The Tao of Later Life

The Tao of Later Life

DAVID "LUCKY" GOFF, PH.D.

ELDER PRESS
Columbus, Ohio

THE TAO OF LATER LIFE

Published by Gatekeeper Press
2167 Stringtown Rd, Suite 109
Columbus, OH 43123-2989
www.GatekeeperPress.com

The cover design, typesetting, and editorial work for this book are entirely the product of the author. Gatekeeper Press did not participate in and is not responsible for any aspect of these elements.

Cover photo: mother of pearl
Cover Design: Mike Jascewski
Interior Design: Gatekeeper Press
Contents: David "Lucky" Goff, PhD.

ISBN (paperback): 9781662932052
eISBN: 9781662932069

A life review
is one of the most important
developmental tasks of later life.

These forays into the past
are a naturally occurring,
universal mental process in older adults.

Only in old age
with the proximity of death
can one truly experience
a personal sense of the entire life cycle.

That makes old age
a unique stage of life
and makes the review of life
at that time equally unique.

Pulitzer-Prize winning gerontologist
Dr. Robert Butler

Contents

Section One

1

. . .

THE EVOLVING ELDER

Introduction

Section 1 – The Evolving Elder

Human nature is stretching out, via a prolonged life, and gaining a bigger picture of what is going on, and this enlarged viewpoint, along with the additional experience longevity provides, alters the view of the human place in Life. Evolution is shining a new light. Life, particularly human life, is not what it used to be! Old age, it turns out, isn't about demise: it is a time for integrating the whole, becoming one with Life.

Autonomy and independence are taking on a new, more complex depth. Aging has revealed a new dimension of what it means to be free. Maturity, especially emotional maturity, is coming to the foreground. By disclosing the freeing value of growth and maturity, the aged have led the way into a world of emotional intelligence. In this world human beings are valued more for who they are, rather than what they do.

Throughout this book I am going to thread my story. It is a story of being slowly torn apart and reassembled by Life. As I write, I am a disabled man who labors at the keyboard, typing with one hand, and seeing with only my one unpatched eye. I am in a wheel chair for my safety. I have a rare form of dysfunctional brain, and as a result, I have no balance. And that is only the beginning of the story.

All of this happened as a result of a hemorrhagic stroke I suffered in 2003. The long aftermath of this event cost me my home, land, family, marriage, career and health. I suffered all these losses when I was 55; now at 67, I can see they were the necessary prelude that helped me realize the paradoxical relationship between loss and gain.

This painful, uncertain period also brought me to a new understanding of Life. With the help of the community of old folks I helped start in 2010, I have learned. Life has created a new way to be old — and even better, a new way to be human.

This is the story about how that new awareness emerged from being reduced, and from a fresh sensitization to Life. Life took from me everything that made up my life, except what is essential (Life's life), and in so doing, showed me something extraordinary. I learned loss is the way Life sensitizes one, hardship enables new faculties, and aging brings a new, larger picture into focus.

My respect for what it means to be human grew. I have found that aging human beings, because they have gone through so much, and because they have been grown by Life, have a greater perspective and a major contribution to make. We all know old people who are not so vibrant. It took a while to discover the difference between old people who were merely older, and old folks on the elder path (see Chapter 2). I see now how Life animates us, and endows some of us, particularly the elders amongst us, with the capacity to experience and express the wonder of it all.

Old age is assumed to be the final stage of life, composed of a steady decline into retirement, frailty, bad health and death. It is seen primarily as a downhill spiral into a largely disabled state. Old people are treated as if all they want to do is retire, withdraw from the world, and roll up and die. They have been assisted in this endeavor, made as comfortable as possible, segregated from others, and dismissed.

Elderhood instead is coming out of the shadows. It is beginning to have a voice of its own. Grey is gaining ground, becoming more than an inspiring story of someone defying the odds. Some of the old have a growing new perspective. They know that something important is going on. They also know that what is emerging isn't yet visible to the masses.

Because life isn't what it is assumed to be, breaking into another phase of it, going within and being exposed to Life's inner ways, is difficult. This difficulty has for too long made the true elder experience hard to accurately perceive.

It is way past time for a new look at the phenomenon of aging, an examination that reveals the ultimate dignity of human life. Such a look also reveals the organic process that is going on. It shows instinctive forces at work, pushing growth and especially integration. The latter stage of life has its own developmental tasks, its own challenges, its own urges. Life is not over. There is a biological form of growth that takes place in latter life, it is mostly inside, and doesn't appear like any form of Life known before. This invisible form of growth, confuses many, and demonstrates that latter human existence is still embedded in Life itself.

Life is not done when the economy doesn't have much use for one. Aging doesn't mean it is all over. In fact, one of the most important gifts of age only comes into view when latter life is reached. A wrinkling, forgetful humanity still has important things to accomplish. This is one of the chief surprises of old age. There is so much to be! There are important, self-chosen tasks that enhance freedom and self-worth, while involving one more deeply in the life of one's great surround.

Our world teeters now, under the weight of great uncertainty. The human drama has taken a turn that seems to threaten all complex life. Life appears to be unbalanced. Everybody capable of reflection is pausing and waiting for a great and uncertain unraveling. Are we poised before evolution or devolution? The new old, especially the elders, are disclosing that Nature is not waiting around to see. The die may, or may not, be cast. But Life is tumbling, as it always has, and the new old are showing up.

Chapter 1
THE THREE MOONS

————

*"What goes on four feet in the morning,
two feet at noon, and three feet in the evening?"*

The riddle of the Sphynx is part of a mythological story, which reveals that human beings have been aware for a long time of the three stages of human life. The knowledge of what life entails, the stops the train of life is bound to make, is known. What those stages actually contain, however, is less well known. And in the case of elderhood, the last of the stages, this is particularly true.

"What goes on four feet in the morning" is childhood. What goes on "two feet at noon" is adulthood. And, what goes on "three feet in the evening" is the aged one. These three stages make up human life, they encapsulate the nature of the human journey from birth to death.

These three stages reveal the arc of human fullness. They capture how meaning unfolds and how humans ripen. And each has its own contributions to make: skip one, and the organism is stunted and malformed. Inherent in the riddle is awareness that knowledge of the wholeness of life is essential to wellbeing.

I am going to briefly describe these three stages in a different way. Each of them is like a moon, exerting a gravitational influence. Each moon exerts a different force, shaping what happens, and pulling for an outcome that conveys the uniqueness, originality, and comprehensiveness of a human being. I do this because I want to highlight the role of natural dynamism in human life. I also want to discuss the third moon as equal to the others, with its own characteristics.

In addition to how life has been prolonged in the last few decades, the nature of later life has dramatically changed. The story of each stage carries familiar elements, but has been substantially altered by the perspective that emerges with a new take on what this final moon is all about. The ancients saw the last stage of being human as dignified decline. So, does much of the modern world, but now it is beginning to show up as ripening, a fulfillment that is unanticipated. This leads to a new, changing story of the three (moons) ages of mankind.

A human life is an integrated whole. There aren't actually any stages. The stage metaphor is just that, a convenient way to try to convey the complex process a human being goes through in a lifetime. The integration of a human into a whole being was implicit in the riddle of life presented by the Sphynx, but for our purposes the details of that integration have changed enormously.

Along with the longevity revolution — the fact that life expectancy has been extended — the most meaningful part of life has shifted. Whereas, once adulthood represented the apex of human life, by virtue of a longer life the later stage of life has been revealed as the one that holds human potentials never seen in large numbers before and, therefore, the stage that offers a higher quality integration. The meaning of human life has been added to.

There is something so precious and innocent about a child. Most of us don't mind the crawling, squalling, questioning disruption, which comes with a curious child. The future shines in the eyes of our offspring. That future is so vulnerable it arouses fierceness in our hearts and a desire to make sure that new life is protected.

This is as it should be. Humans come into life in a very vulnerable state. Nature has seen fit to shape human consciousness slowly by making human offspring take years to develop. This enables their brains to grow large and complex, and also gives time for the important transmission of culture, the experiential manual of how we do things. Childhood has a lot of important steps in growth that enable a newborn to become a viable, ongoing, autonomous being.

The complexity of the move from the incredibly vulnerable newborn to strapping young being, capable of re-producing, deserves to be a stage of its own. There are unique features of this movement, which are presumed to only happen in childhood. Notice I said presumed, because this is where the familiar story shifts. Childhood's innocence is going to come back later. The fact that it does, reveals that this attribute is more enduring and resilient than presently thought. Child-like attributes, like play, have a larger meaning.

Developmental patterns, like those associated with childhood, are plastic, and change occurs in dramatically unforeseen ways further on in life. The stage of childhood prepares one for life, but not fully, and this becomes most evident later when Life asks more of one. Childhood is a necessary precursor, but many of the coping mechanisms one learns in childhood must be given up to live fully and adapt to a more complex perception of life.

In the big scheme of things, childhood is seen as the way one becomes capable of functionally entering the world. Rudimentary skills are enough to get one into the flow of the game, but are not enough to grasp all of the subtleties of play. Survival is essentially a focus of development, but what one is surviving for, in most cases, is determined later in life.

Childhood is seen as a valuable time of preparation. The first stage of life is devoted to ensuring that the child is readied to be a viable adult. Adult life is seen as the apex of life, and childhood is organized around it. This makes sense. It follows the time-honored belief that maximum physical competency represents the greatest achievement for the community.

This, however, is no longer a simple truth. When we come to examine the qualities of the new Elderhood, a picture arises that complicates the notion that adulthood is the best part of the human journey. It is likely that the new features of Elderhood warrant some re-organization. Life seems to be providing a stimulus that prompts change.

There is a very interesting transitional phase (a time between the worlds), which has complexities that don't appear earlier in childhood, and are frowned on if they appear later in adulthood. This period, we refer to as adolescence, and generally associate it with becoming an adult. It is a unique part of childhood, which is complex and troublesome. It is an awkward time. Hormones are raging. Individual, and culture, are struggling to find accommodation.

I'm underscoring adolescence, because there is a later transformation (another time between the worlds), which is similar to it, but very different. Adolescence opens the door to adulthood. There is currently no generally accepted name for the unique form of shift, corresponding with adolescence, that opens the door to old age. More complex, and more rewarding, this opening, echoes adolescence, and offers greater maturity for those who pass through it.

But, before we humans get there, we have to undergo a most arduous and confusing threshold we have named adolescence. It contains within it a painful and upsetting time between. In the case of each human there is a period, sometimes brief, sometimes not so brief, where Life delivers one to the next stage, but not before changing one.

This period is often marked in indigenous cultures with some kind of initiation. Generally speaking, here in the western industrial world, we don't have such clear social indicators. People suffer this absence. They still make the journey. Adolescence is a moment of suspension where, whether we like it or not, we are thrust into the adult world. Adulthood in modern cultures is assumed to happen with age, and it is often an involuntary experience that happens alone. It is like an approaching storm, offering only the dimmest recognition about upcoming responsibilities while taking one on a careening ride.

Some people come through intact, with a sense of themselves and knowledge about how they want to serve. They are a minority. Even with so much going for them, they still have to establish themselves, and if being authentic means living outside the mainstream, they may never really get to be freely themselves. Adolescence is pretty much a crapshoot with only a few actually moving toward their authentic potential. This has implications for individual and society alike, as does the return of these issues later in life.

Some time in our teenage years, a second moon comes over the horizon. When it does, one is thrust into adolescent turmoil. In some alchemical way, hormones mix with responsibility, the desire to know oneself, and the societal pull towards fitting in. Young people become citizens.

Adulthood, for too many, is a way to conform and become acceptable, leaving behind the dreams that made one unique. The trade-off for financial viability has a Faustian quality; people give up so much to acquire the economic power that seems to assure life. Work is too often what confers status and wellbeing. People grow obsessed by business, activity, and doing. Thus, the ubiquitous party question: what do you do?

It is strange to realize that development doesn't stop with finding —whatever one does. Nature seems to be interested in more than becoming economically productive. Somehow, the urge to grow goes on despite the norms of an urbane, busy, active life. What takes place is a lot of culturally-induced activity, providing the illusion of personal growth and progress, while in fact most of the growth takes place within, in the interior.

People marry, have kids, divorce, change careers, and consult life coaches, therapists, and a variety of other experts, trying to appease the inner unrest that accompanies modern life. All of this looks like growth, but only some of it is. Some get really depressed and anxious. Adulthood carries a price, which is often considered the dues one has to pay to acquire the riches of life. Since adulthood is seen as the apex of life, there is a lot of pressure to achieve, and a fear of what will happen if one doesn't.

One lives under the influence of this moon for a long time, maybe 30 or 40 years. The tendency to believe that this is it, the sum of life, is pretty great. Acquiring the fruits of life seems to be what everybody is up to. So, one goes along, dimly aware that aging (and maturing) is changing the nature of the game. Too many people count on being the exception, having access to some technological breakthrough that will rescue them.

The rat race prevents one from looking up to see clearly the approach of old age. The level of entrenchment is very great. So much so, there is a kind of nostalgia for the earlier days, the times when it was unclear where one was going, a moment when there was time for friends. That all seems to be in the past — over — the needs of future generations are all that matter now. Adulthood is about ensuring the future by activity. It is a well-intentioned use of life-energy that leads one deeper into believing this is the only moment that matters.

Some people look forward to a time when they are on the sidelines, when they are financially comfortable, and no one is telling them what to do. Retirement, to these few, represents a kind of reward. Some say retirement is a dirty word, some a just reward, some say it comes with a sense of being put out to pasture, to some it is being forgotten, and to a few it is the happiest they have ever been. But to all, it is the rising of a third, unfamiliar, and semi-expected moon.

When this moon comes over the horizon it causes people to quake with uncertainty. To the aging folks alive today, this moment is like when ancient people first beheld an eclipse: there are many dreadful stories about what is happening. A natural event is taking place. It will not hurt us; in fact, the fact that it is occurring enhances our chances for living more accurately in this world. In our present world this rising portends an unknown universe. This is a scary and liberating event.

A major part of the difficulty people have coming to terms with old age is the reaction to the appearance of this moon. When this moon rises, the widespread reaction to it is reduces the chances that many will ever grasp the opportunities it brings.

The last phase of human life has mostly been considered a time when one limps across the finish line. Maybe one is seen (if one is lucky) as wiser, but usually one is seen as broken down and physically spent. This obscures the real advance that comes with this stage of life. The penchant (that most humans have because they tend to see things from earlier stages of life) is to miss the incredible move inward — from doing to being. Inner life is emphasized at this stage. One in early life is easily swayed by the desire to be like somebody, or something outside of one self. Life in this final stage pulls a big switcheroo. It diminishes us — limiting functioning, and making it difficult to move easily toward external things, while enhancing the capacity to integrate inner things.

The last stage of life suffers from the very human tendency to view everything through an earlier lens. In this case, the burgeoning inner life of old people is viewed through the eyes of younger people who can see the surface of things. From this viewpoint, aging looks like physical decline. However, something really different is going on. The aging ones are being put through a shift that, by and large, is not expected, and is unprepared for.

In addition to the difficulty associated with moving inward in a world that has always emphasized externalities, there is another aspect of increasing age that causes trouble. This is loss. There is something paradoxical about the experience of loss, which makes the benefits it confers non-obvious, and subject to the misinterpretation of others.

There are a host of losses that come with later life, too many to enumerate, but losses typically associated with old age are emotional hits that take a while to integrate. The loss of vigor, health, prestige, influence, economic wellbeing, and productive capacity, all change the picture, making it look grim indeed. What is going on is subtle, not really visible. Life is putting the individual through a difficult transition, from someone who was somebody, by the signs of the world, to somebody who finds their value inside. This is a rigorous development that happens within and is, therefore, not really obvious.

Add to what has just been described — a realization that as one advances in age — one enters more fully into the land of death. This is the ultimate loss. Old age looks disturbing to many people because, by and large, folks have not really come to terms with death. While the studies of the attitudes and experiences of the old, show that death is not such a fearsome prospect, those entering, or about to enter this realm, tend to fear the worst. This reflects how deeply cultural anxiety about death distresses so many. This tendency, in turn, affects the way aging is perceived.

This transition is difficult. It is even more complex and demanding than the earlier difficulties associated with adolescence. An old person coming upon this stage of Life (Grandolescence) is all too often influenced by fear and/or treated as if they are the carrier of a terrible, infectious disease. This makes the likelihood of a successful transition rare; which in turn, tends to verify the assumptions that prevail. Old age is viewed like dropping off the edge of the world.

Instead of all of these dire assumptions, elderhood is positively bursting with good qualities, which people currently have difficulty reaching. The amazing thing, and the thing that suggests that a change is coming, is that some people make this transition anyway.

These rare folks know that getting old offers a view of the whole of human times, and one's place within that big picture. They are also the ones who have come home to themselves, and offer a new vision of human possibility. The best of life is actually saved for last — the integration that takes place in the latter years. It is a gift from the cosmos that changes everything.

The metaphor of the three moons represents an attempt to describe the vital natural forces at work in shaping a human life. In an attempt to describe the natural forces at work, the gravitational effects of celestial bodies seem apt. There is something about shifting from an external perspective to an internal one that is characteristic of old age, and is difficult to perceive in our time. Doing so, makes the integrative force more explicit, shows how beholden we still are to Nature.

Elderhood is the phase of life where this integrative force is strongest. All of the benefits of this stage stem from a desire, evidently spurred on by Nature, to bring all of it together, to actualize what Nature has started. The influence of Nature in this development is too important to ignore. Old people, particularly elders, are boosted in their development by this invisible, elemental force.

Despite the taint of fear and prejudice, old age endures and is growing. For elders, something else a whole lot more extraordinary is happening. When it does, Life is affirmed. It becomes us, or more accurately, we become it. It is in our old age, when it is possible to discover that Life has been with us throughout our journey.

Chapter 2
GRANDOLESCENCE:
A SHIFTING PERSPECTIVE

I can't emphasize enough that, when the moon of old age comes over the horizon, most people are not prepared for the magnitude of change that they are about to undergo. This shift is tantamount to becoming a parent and never grasping until the child comes what parenting actually entails.

Like the ancients viewing an eclipse for the first time, a lot of fear gets stirred up. It takes a while to grasp the new reality that has just come into view. Life has other plans for us, and it is ruthlessly and impeccably carrying them out. I will describe that shift. I've even given it a name, *grandolescence,* to make it more memorable,

This is a monumental, new change. It has its initiatory ordeals but leads to a significantly good outcome. Associating it with the grandness of Life motivated me. So, did the desire to remind everybody that *changing* is part of the *becoming* that characterizes human nature. The reference to adolescence in the name intentionally refers to the changes one has to go through to be a mature human. Thus, grandolescence.

The heart of grandolescence, or the transition from adulthood, is fraught with elements that make this shift anything but straightforward. It is like stepping through a looking glass. The non-obvious challenge (along with a significant benefit) is that the looking glass is within. Another element that makes this transition non-intuitive and difficult is that it involves a loss of control. Nature is driving this shift. It isn't voluntary.

With losses come the gains. The gains, however, are not obvious at first. In fact, they are obscured by the assumptions that prevail in earlier life. The research on centenarians (people 100 or older), the fastest growing segment of the population, shows that wellbeing for old folks depends upon escaping the dictates of cultural assumptions. The process of escaping, at first, feels like being cut off from all which one knows. The new freedom that comes with this change of Life is often unwelcome, disorienting and threatening.

These difficulties make the transition from adulthood arduous. They also make this journey profoundly altering. What emerges from it is a renewed human being, one who is less self-oriented, while paradoxically being *more* self-oriented.

A painful dimension of the shift has to do with a radical reorientation of self. For many, the losses (place, status, prestige, health, influence, financial wellbeing, and sometimes autonomy) that attend this form of coming of age are significant, overwhelming and mesmerizing. Add to this the fact that one's culture considers these losses tragic. The apparently tragic aspect captures awareness and gives the impression that aging has victimized one. It seems that injustice has occurred. This is confounding and often consumes one's attention, while an inexorable change is taking place within.

Life is executing a move away from the kind of external-orientation that prevails in modern day-to-day efforts to a focus within, to locating one's sense of self in who one *is* rather than in what one *does*. A move away from doing to being is happening. It is a shift that takes place within.

The hub-bub that is caused by all of the losses, along with the apparent injustice, distracts one, providing a disguise, obscuring the fact that the nature of life is changing things from within. The scale of balance is shifting, identity is eroding, and Life is once more transforming our nature — underscoring the fact that we are creatures of the Universe, not solely our own.

The truth is that we are being shifted, sometimes against our will, sometimes confusingly, mostly mystifyingly. The difficulty we humans have making this shift isn't just our own fault — this transformation is plainly difficult! Ageism is a big factor, the fear and ignorance of most of the world's cultures is significant; these prejudices make this arduous natural transition all the harder. But ageism alone does not account for how challenging it is. Nature has concocted a passageway into a greater life that is as trying as any birth. Grandolescence strips us before it delivers us to the next stage of Life.

This is the place where my story is relevant. It reveals why I might have this outlook. Basically, Life killed off who I used to be, and permanently changed me, sensitizing me to the challenges and opportunities associated with living as an altered being. The process of being killed off was painful and confusing.

I had a hemorrhagic stroke, which was followed, even before I could begin recovering from the stroke, with a rare brain problem that my doctors had never seen, and couldn't diagnose, or treat. I was dying. I was left alone to face a gradually failing life that seemed to be leading to a certain death. Does that sound familiar? It should, because that is exactly what the dark side of grandolescence looks and feels like.

As I went down, I had the normal amount of self-pity. I lamented and wondered why. I lost functioning, my home, marriage and family, career, health and wellbeing. Life took my life, and all I was left with was rubble. After 4 years of living like a terminal patient (with a planning horizon that never exceeded 24 hours) and gradually losing more functioning, I gave up all hope. I felt helpless. There was no way out. I began planning to become a vegetable with no control of my bodily functions and a terrible awareness of what was happening. I began to think of assisted suicide.

It is unlikely that many people will have to go through the kind of dramatic, all-consuming uncertainty I did. I began emerging, coming back to life when, in my final surrender, I realized that what I thought of as *my* life was actually Life's life. It turned out that this change in my perspective enabled me to survive and return to this life, disabled, but feeling lucky. I have been given a fresh chance at life, with a renewed perspective. The journey back from the edge was not easy, but it was accompanied with the realization that Life is actively managing me.

It has been awhile since I was thrust so completely into the maw of death. In that time, I've become more aware of the machinations of Life. I've come to a new appreciation of Life's impact on humans. As I have gradually integrated my experience, I've come to see that each of us is intended by Life, and there is nothing random about the difficulties Life asks us to bear. The challenges Life poses educate and shape us, drawing out of us our own uniqueness, freeing us to be ourselves, and to celebrate life as extensions of the Life force.

Being so thoroughly decimated made it possible for me to see a larger picture, and to become a larger person. Now, I've come to see a variation of the same thing in grandolescence. It is a natural process, a bittersweet gift of Life, exacting from us our superfluities and gifting us with our own unique selves, the snowflakes of light within. Grandolescence is too valuable an experience to be buried in ageism and misinterpretation.

The experience of being alone left me to seek and rely on myself, to go within, to discover the resources that made survival more likely. Grandolescence does the same. The emotional hits that come with loss are accurately aimed, customized to be extraordinarily personal, to heighten awareness of how alone one is so that one must find their identity within.

A renewed inner life enables the fresh take on existence which old age brings. Again, the rigor of this change is awesome. It is no wonder one often hears, "Old age isn't for the faint-hearted." Grandolescence is involuntary, involves loss, and provokes internal awareness. By and large, these are not welcome developments.

There is no insurance policy or retirement account that will forestall the ravages of time. Life has an inexorable trait. Everything that can be lost, will be. This isn't a popular realization. These losses hurt, and they also serve to mature us. No wonder old age is viewed unfavorably. Luckily, loss isn't the end of the story. But it is an essential part of it. The journey into greater human maturity means coming to accept loss as a natural part of Life.

Life is puncturing the illusion that it isn't in charge. There is a growth-dance associated with aging, which one is being invited to. The invitation is gilded with disappointment and loss. The call to maturity doesn't come in a form that is easily accepted. But accept it we must.

Growing larger often means surrendering the very things that once conferred a sense of identity. Rather painfully, this can mean old laments about how others have treated one. For instance, I know someone who has had to give up her feeling of being abandoned. Whether or not she was abandoned as a child, at the age of 60 this aspect of her experience couldn't be allowed to define her life anymore.

For her, maturing meant giving up an old sensitivity. This sensitivity had become a requirement of relationship, one that hobbled her. She could not afford to leave her wellbeing in the hands of others. They consistently let her down. So, for her, this meant facing the prospect of never having what she needed from others, and giving up trying to get it from them anymore. She turned, of necessity, to herself, inward, to the one that remained, for what she could give to herself. Letting go, for her, meant gaining a new ally, turning in for the one who remained.

Letting go is a challenging part of growing older. It is a particularly elder skill. Letting go is not intuitively obvious. It is a form of self-sacrifice, a choice that has the paradoxical impact of enabling further growth. It involves the giving up of old hopes (particularly of others) in favor of new abilities (of one's own). Learning that this practice, letting go, has a maturing effect, is a by-product of losing. This educative aspect of losing characterizes grandolescence. Without feeling the ravages and the emotional burn of loss, a gain cannot occur. This is a natural part of wisdom that cannot be integrated without loss.

Still, this form of loss, even if it is voluntary, is not very appetizing. It rankles those who are attached to ideas of invulnerability, freedom from ambivalence, and invincibility. These seemingly adult attributes, extolled by societies mad for control, serve only to delay and obfuscate the on-set of the natural maturing process. Life alters our wrong-headed attachments and unceremoniously sets us on a better, albeit more difficult, path. That difficulty is exacerbated by our beliefs.

Grandolescence is the beginning. It introduces loss, but also contains gain. It acquaints us with a new world, a place where paradox reigns. Grasping the world anew reintroduces us to our own reborn innocence and calls for a kind of beginner's mind. Grandolescence introduces changes that don't come easily in a world that has always emphasized knowing and being in charge. Discovering the humbling, but freeing truth — that the more one knows, the less one knows — is hard, but the doorway to the land of paradox opens.

All of this happens: internal and external landscapes change, the rules of living alter, and Life and mortality become more obvious. Grandolescence marks the beginning of becoming grandly human, of discovering that Life is still enchanting, and that existence is a privilege. The moon coming over the horizon is an integrative moon, which paradoxically removes the superfluous (causing some initial discomfort), retrains us, and reveals more clearly what really matters about Life. The process is elegant, even profound, but while one is in it, grandolescence is confounding.

Grandolescence is also very humbling. With it comes a growing realization of one's mortality. There is nothing so humbling as recognizing that despite how one has lived, death still awaits. This, increasingly, is a more undeniable fact. Death is all around now.

A big part of the losses that accompany this phase is the death of loved ones. Many are confronted with the loss and/or caretaking of parents, spouses and friends. When this happens, a new or deeper awareness comes about. Time is growing shorter. Life is not going to last forever.

The realization of the approach of termination galvanizes one. It leads to the creation of bucket lists, travel plans, and renewed relationships with family, friends, and others. Surprisingly, the proximity of death, also tends to lead to a deepening of one's relationship with oneself. Just as spiritual matters become more important, so does reflection upon the nature of one's own life. An approaching death shines a bright light on all the uncertainties that have accompanied one's existence. It is a sobering and liberating time. One is faced with limitation and is thereby freed in a way that nothing else could do. The realization of the inevitability of death is one of the greatest gifts of grandolescence, because it renews the emphasis upon Life.

Death is sobering. It tends to focus one's attention. It is also refreshingly clarifying. It is a favor to us. It may look like the end, reducing one's chances of living fully; but because it is the end, it actually enhances our chances of living more fully. Paradoxically, the end of life brings out more of the desire to live life to its fullest, to be alive while one still can. Death is a ripening agent.

The fatal end is what ensures a deeper engagement with being here. Death rouses us, deepening our desire, firing up our grief, and focusing us upon the unfinished business of living. It is the way that death twists us, which brings the paradoxical nature of grandolescence and later, elder life, into view. There are gifts to be had in elder life that are not available earlier. These gifts accompany losses. The limitations that come with old age are all empowering developments, which can be relied upon to deepen one's engagement with the miracle of Life.

Aging alone doesn't confer anything. Aging thickens the broth; it moves everything, closing some doors and opening others. It raises a storm of fresh potential, but the latency aroused, while evenly distributed, is not evenly accepted.

We all know people who are merely old. They deserve respect, but their inflexibility defines them. Merely old people are the majority of old folks, they live a life governed by the past, and they are not actualizers of the new capabilities emerging with true elders. Nature strikes where it will. Old people deserve a break. They are our veterans. But there are some, a minority, who experience something fresh. They are hard to see because they are as grey as their peers. They are subject to the same kind of prejudicial treatment. But there is an important difference between a merely older person and the new elder.

This difference is enormously important. So much so, that I'm going to spend the bulk of this section differentiating the two. The advantages that come via elder awareness are only available to us in any widespread way, if the differences between what is merely old and what is truly new, is perceptible. Defining the merely old helps define the new elder.

Who are elders, after all, and how are they different from the merely old? An easy and quick response to that question is that elders still have some life in front of them, while the merely old are finished and waiting to die. This quick response, however, conveys the impression that one is easily told from another. This is not true.

While the merely old tend to be more rigid and less interested in surprises, the two have much in common, which can make telling them apart challenging. For one thing, cultural assumptions about aging make all old people look alike. Many of the old are simply invisible. Elders, like other old people, are frequently treated mistakenly, as if they were over the hill, declining, and basically worthless. The youthful orientation that prevails in this culture obscures old people — and robs them all of dignity, identity, and uniqueness.

The old all chafe from this treatment, and our culture misses making an important distinction. When this happens, a disabling cost befalls us all. The elderly are treated badly, the gifts that come through elders are missed, and everyone else fails to know what we humans are capable of. The old pay the heaviest price, but those who are younger suffer from not knowing what Life really offers. The best of Life is saved for last.

The merely old are those who have found comfort in familiar, life-draining ruts. They are captives of resignation. They have internalized most all of the ageist assumptions, and given in. Elders, on the other hand, are fighting their way out of stereotypes, ruts, and the life-nullifying messages that are prevalent. For them, there is a creative impulse that governs their engagement with life. They are in the process of discovering their true nature.

Humans are creatures of habit. We are not above doing the same old repetitive thing that once worked. Like a rat in a maze, it is very human to seek rewards we know. The habitual becomes a yoke that ties us to the past. We create and live in ruts of our own devising. This normal human trait, however, has big implications.

To go further we have to go beyond ourselves. This means abandoning all of the success strategies that have carried us this far. Becoming a beginner, a new being unshielded by what one has learned, is not easy or desirable. Choosing to begin again, to walk naked into the glare of the light, doesn't come easily. It is amazing some people do it! Life can be insistent; some are admittedly dragged into growth. But the benefits of hardship, with a feeling of something compelling stirring inside, impel some to ripen.

Elders have extraordinary experiences of transcending themselves. They go beyond the ruts, old ways, and attachments that have previously defined them. They have the experience, not always voluntary, of having given up control. They know that death awaits them, and that it can take many forms. For them, returning to old behaviors is a form of death.

We are an extremely adaptable species, with enormous potential. The challenge we face, however, individually and as a species, is matching our growth and development with our historical circumstances. Elders are very adept at this.

While we are living, we are subject to the influences of our environment. In the earliest stages of life others are very influential; later on, it is primarily our desire, our willingness, that determines what we make of what Life presents us with. In each case growth is a kind of dance.

Our steps determine the quality of our dance, but Life, as our partner, leads. Life leads, but how we follow is totally idiosyncratic, unique, and up to us. The dance proceeds according to a combination of moves between the two. Our responses to Life customize us, making us more or less mature. This is the privilege of being human, the contribution we humans make to creation, and it is always coupled with the ministrations of Life.

The lament that new parents often express, "that there is no manual," is actually true for the whole of human life. All of us are confronted with the difficult task of determining for ourselves how much we are willing to use the adaptive capacities given to each of us. This is a matter of choice. And, it is always a challenge, which separates the merely old from the wrinkled and grey beginners.

The journey from childhood through adulthood to elderhood is a wild ride. It has many turning points, many ways to get off on another track. This is the primary reason that out of a growing number of old people only some of them are elders. Simply surviving the twists and turns of Life, though worthy of respect, isn't the same as thriving with a growing complex awareness. This awareness takes shape through weathering many storms, through experiencing heartaches, and choosing to live one's life for the sake of the whole. Aging is an organic journey, but not everybody learns to thrive. Life for the true elder is a miracle that has implications for all.

Elders are more self-possessed, more interested in others, less emotionally reactive and judgmental, more compassionate, and eager to serve the larger communities they feel themselves to be part of. They are motivated more from the inside out rather than the outside in. They are more self-confrontive and treat themselves and Life better. They know what their purpose is. Elders are humble; they know they are older and wiser because of life experiences and hardships. They are who they are because Life made them that way. They are the ones who have learned the alchemical trick of turning lemons into joyous lives.

This kind of development is rare, because too few know of it, and because we currently have no cultural supports for it. Elders pass amongst us, like most old people, ignored, unseen, and mis-valued. They have actualized some of our human potentials. They could reveal a lot about what we are capable of. But caught up in a consensus trance, brought on by our penchant for valuing the young and staying economically active, we miss what they have to offer.

Elders are making it through the maturational change points that bring out our human potential. They are the ones who have turned the travails of Life into something that can serve us all. They face the difficulties of living, and they find the ways to convert those difficulties into assets. We are all going to lose capabilities, to need others, to be sick and infirm, to die. Maybe we could learn what elders seem to know — that being human is a challenging blessing.

Elders are most easily distinguished from the merely old through relationship. Elders have hallmark relational capabilities. These cannot be faked. They are a product of growth and development. Simply put, if you are interested in knowing if someone is an elder, and not merely elderly, spend a little time with them. Depth is obvious. You'll know very quickly if you are experiencing an elder. Presence, interest, and availability are the signs.

There is a host of distinguishing factors that sets old people apart, but they are all disguised by one similarity; that in our ageist culture, prevents most people from identifying elders. Both are old, wrinkled, grey and losing their faculties. The old are treated democratically alike; they are uniformly de-valued.

Both elders and merely old folks are needed. Each carries an important awareness. But elder awareness and the kind of wisdom available to it is important to us because it carries our prospects. The future of humanity is unfolding right now. As elders delve into the unknown, the orbit of our kind is expanding. Tomorrow's possibilities are coming into view. So, it is important to know that true elders are around and to know what they are capable of.

Grandolescence marks the onset of a long period of fluidity. It starts with changes that feel and appear tragic. Real losses accompany this change of Life. That isn't the end of the story, but in the early part of these changes Life alters the way we feel about ourselves.

Grandolescence threatens our self-images and casts us into unknown waters. Life thrusts us beyond ourselves, and then asks us to become even more. Some are simply over their heads, some don't want to be asked to be more, some are unable to surrender control, and some, a rare minority, thrive in a new way.

Grandolescence, by virtue of stripping down most people, is making possible a new life. Some of us are drafted into it; it feels so intense that few of us would have elected to experience it. Thankfully, Life in its greater wisdom initiates us anyway.

This seems like a propitious place to return to my story. Remember, at age 55 Life pruned me. It took and dismembered me. All of the ways I thought of and valued myself were stripped away. I was unable to move, talk, and relate. I started recovering, or so my doctors and I thought. Instead, a rare brain syndrome set in, one that slowly took away my remaining functions and left me expecting to die. The process was deadly slow. It took four years and during that time, since no one could help me, I lost all hope.

I was bereft. I lost so much I couldn't even tell, at any given moment, what I was grieving. Was it my marriage, home, family, career, or health? I didn't know. All I knew was that I'd been hit by a terrible blizzard of loss. I spent many years in this condition, expecting to eventually die. I didn't, and because I didn't, I learned many things. While waiting to die, I was blessed (though I didn't know it at the time) with a pile of losses that seemed to convey to me how defective, unloved, and lost I was. The thoroughness of my losses were mesmerizing; I just couldn't see anything else. I even dreamed I was a storm victim — I searched despondently through the rubble of my house.

It turned out that what remained saved me. I didn't know that would be the case, but I reached the place where I knew that looking as intently as I was at what I had lost was killing me. I was reduced to a slab of meat. I was only waiting for the final moment. But it never came. I didn't have the physical capacity to help myself, but I realized, for the sake of my mind, that I had to look at something beyond my losses. So, without the benefit of hope, because I was desperate and lost, I began looking around for something else to pay attention to.

I don't know when I hit on what remained. But slowly, agonizingly slowly, I was able to pull my attention away from my large, compelling pile of losses to the rather humble pile of what remained. That move, which took over a year to pull off, saved me. I didn't know it at the time, but a lot more remained than I knew. I've been discovering in the intervening years just how much.

This move took time; it allowed me not only to live, but it began a process of discovering what the losses had obscured. There were other factors that have allowed me to thrive and feel as lucky as I do today, but suffice it to say, that *shifting my gaze from the losses to what remained* enabled me to find the gains that accompanied those losses. This experience cued me in to what grandolescence potentiates in each of us. The gains are a result, a commensurate development, of the losses. One accompanies the other.

Each element of ourselves that is stripped from us has a corresponding development — a gain of self. Life shifts us —altering who we are — not for our sakes, nor in our own comforting time — because something else is more important than our expectations. This something else looks to me like evolution.

People who have survived other scary things, like the death of a loved one, illness, financial ruin, being laid off, or other losses, know that something happens. Life changes. But, most of us have to be re-awakened, have to be reintroduced to our own new capabilities.

This is why I will spend so much energy talking about the importance of community in elder lives. Rubbing shoulders with others who have undergone grandolescence re-awakens old people to the gifts that aging has brought them. The move from independence, where everybody is alone, to interdependence, where everybody is connected, is unfolding. This move is so substantial and unexpected that it takes others to fully realize. The world has changed in ways others confirm.

Grandolescence introduces one to an era of one's life that, as mentioned, is paradoxical, and is characterized by the fascinating combination of two opposites: loss and gain. They arrive linked, though it often takes time to see how they are related. The loss can happen long before the gain. The inner world is shifting. As one gets used to the outer world of flux, a light goes on within. More subtle changes are on the way.

Because we live in a world that does not recognize grandolescence, most people entering this phase will blame themselves for the losses they endure. All is not lost, however. Nature is on the prowl, looking for ways of converting heartaches into sensitivities, lost or broken identities into new lives, and physical limitations into relationship skills. The loss of hearing may lead to listening more intently. The loss of memory may generate living happily in the present moment. The proximity of death will educate one. Hopelessness makes one more malleable. Reduction sets in. Life calls all of us, but few respond. I know. Leaning into the losses, and finding the way to the gains, is an exacting path. One that is strangely predictable in its unpredictable nature.

There is an invisible passageway that confronts us all. It is like a sifter, a natural strainer. The rising of the moon of old age, brings on this natural filter. In too many cultures this is seen as the end of the story. Instead, something new is happening. In some unforeseen way something predictable is turning into something unpredictable. By past standards this development is implausible. Rationality and logic say only so many things can happen at this juncture of Life. Life, however, doesn't concur. Some old people are slipping the noose of expectations and going further. Unbelievable as it may seem, evolution is cooking up a new scenario for our kind — it's an initiation brought on by Life.

Grandolescence is like a permeable wall. It initially slows one, not entirely, but gradually and effectively. It doesn't stop the motions of life, but it does change the meaning that life holds. The hardship this phase of Life introduces, drives one in, where the search for integration kicks into high gear. Greying and losing functioning are the hallmarks of this change, just like the advent of pubic hair and youthful vigor are the hallmarks of adolescence. And, just as before, how one responds to this change determines the quality of what is to follow. Resistance is futile. The pressure of Life, found in the aging process, is having its way with us.

Grandolescence isn't an overnight transition. It takes time. The losses seldom come all at once. Adolescence takes about five years to unfold (from 13 to 18). The simplicities of childhood eventually give way to the new complexities of adulthood. Grandolescence is similar, but it takes longer. The complexity of this shift is much greater. Therefore, starting when Life determines, the shift into old age takes anywhere from 8 to 20 years.

During that time a striking transformation is occurring. Typically, this move starts out with dramatic lifestyle changes that seem to be imposed from without, and proceed via changes that are brought about from within. A new vocabulary starts to emerge. "Acceptance," "surrender" "letting go" convey experience with loss. The pattern of transition goes from defoliation to exfoliation. Eventually people begin leaning into the changes taking place. Some have succeeded in shifting their gaze, seeing these changes not as difficulties but as opportunities. For a small minority of old folks, life becomes about actualizing potential and becoming Life incarnate.

Grandolescence is a gift of Nature. It is a ripening ordeal. True initiation has always looked harsh, but it brings out the best in us. Life provides the necessary and timely challenges. To become a fully ripe human being involves grief. The hardships it takes, the losses that are endured, enable wisdom.

Chapter 3
REDUCTION — THE ELDER PATH

———

When the third moon comes over the horizon a transformation begins. As that moon rises a further arduous path materializes. The rather paradoxical losses/gains of grandolescence become a more permanent and consistent state. Loss and gain continue, only now these changes are more predictable. Late life is governed by reduction.

Reduction is a paradoxical process, which bears some resemblance to grandolescence, but is more final, complete and pervasive. It happens to everybody. And, reduction never ends. It is a pattern that includes shrinking, but pairs it with a most amazing deepening. Reduction is much like the process of sauce-making of the same name. While cooking a good sauce one "reduces" it by increasing the heat to burn off the diluting inessentials. The process of reduction diminishes the quantity and brings out innate qualities (what's within).

Through a similar form of alchemy, Nature uses the losses of aging to bring out depth and character. The formula is diminishment creating depth — and if cooperated with, this pattern brings incredible new meaning and capacities. Our response to the rigors of reduction, determines the quality we bring into our elder years. So, the focus upon diminishment that defines the later years is understandable, as physical capabilities are changing. Because of the inability to see beyond the surface, important new capabilities arising from within are all too easily overlooked.

This creates a distortion that is perpetuated daily. The old in particular suffer, because they don't often know their own potential, nor what lies within. Younger folks suffer, too, because they also don't know the potentials they embody, nor do they have any recognition that depth lies within, and that it offers them the prospect of a better life. The habitual treatment of old age as a disability adds to the fear of later life, and entirely misses the real movement of Life.

Reduction isn't just a word. It is a series of simplifications that Life imposes on one until the final moment. Old age brings with it what looks and feels like a litany of complaints. These range from physical problems to issues with family, economic concerns. and isolation. There is a loss of mobility and social connection. In essence it seems like Life is dragging one downhill. And, then one dies. The final moon looks like a bad trip.

The typical experience of the old, is summed up by shrinking. This isn't a product of being analyzed by a psycho-professional, it is the change of stature that gravity imposes. One just gets smaller. Life reduces one's physical body, removing a lot of capabilities, re-casting one into a more vulnerable physical state. Vitality, bones, senses, energy and wellbeing are all affected. To the old this turn in the plotline suggests the final scene.

The losses built into aging are hard to take. Without any alternative notion of what is going on, it is easy to subscribe to the prevailing assumption that the story is all over. So, there is not only a physical kind of diminishment going on, there is a simultaneous diminution of options. The old one is on a shrinking path with shrinking options that lead to an inevitable end. It is hard to believe otherwise. Industries, retirement plans, and media all reinforce this idea, so the old one is subject to being shrunk out of existence by shrinking expectations.

Elderhood is about integration. The story of a lifetime not only becomes clearer, but in some cases, morphs into something else. To do this, natural influences take place. These influences defy cultural expectations, and thus make old age a place of struggle. The shrinking expectations that prevail on one side, conflict with the innate desire for the freedom of self-actualization on the other.

Currently, the inner world that becomes so present as one ages is invisible. This has the effect of cultural denial, a mass disbelief in the realities of old age. Old people are buffeted around by the dissonance this causes. It is hard enough dealing with a radical life change. Add to that, the wrong assumptions that are made everywhere. This forces those who have the desire to live fully, and to be authentic and present, into a kind of counter-cultural position. They are left to inquire within without supports, while trying to throw off the baggage of expectations that prevent them from being themselves.

Staying with the rigors that are innate to becoming old, the integrative thrust of this new moon means that the process of forging a meaningful life has come to a very dramatic and essential era. All that has come before, has led up to this time. Possibilities must be assessed. Some of them must be surrendered, some of them remain to be actualized, some surprises are met. One must decide if they are finished yet or not. All along the way culture, in the form of loved ones, family, friends, and strangers, whispers bad — and life-nullifying — advice.

The primary goal of the reductive process is to aid integration. It is a kind of clarifying thrust. In the meantime, however, the typical old person is having their life turned inside out and, furthermore, outside in. There is a paradoxical gauntlet to run, one that isn't even supposed to exist. But it does. And with the advent of the third moon, the moon of Elderhood, there are many such moments.

Death with its solving justice lurks nearby, clarifying what matters, and giving us incentive to finish sculpting ourselves. The new integrative force that comes into life has a purpose. It is to prompt us to get on with life, and to do so for the sake of authentic uniqueness.

The Universe wants diversity as much as it wants unity. Life gives to those that comply. There is a deeper kind of unique authenticity available to the impetuous ones who live up to what Life is asking.

Essentializing isn't just about life being over. It is a mode of clarifying and summing up. Life becomes clearer, and in so doing becomes more miraculous, sending some old folks into another orbit. Reduction is Life altering one's viewpoint. For most of us that simply means getting clearer on what we have been up to in this world; but for some of us, a minority of old folks, it is an introduction to a new set of possibilities. In both cases reduction, in paradoxical fashion, provides a new form of clarifying energy. This, for some, is an unexpected gain, which offers a new perspective, renewed clarity, and a life that has fresh new attributes. For the very few, the elders-in-training, this is the call of the wild, the chance to be one with the life force.

Take "stuff" for instance. Throughout the earlier part of life, one gathers everything that one feels is essential. This accumulation of things includes household items, tools, playthings, sports stuff, papers, artwork, photos, hobby items, sentimental things, kitchenware and vehicles. As one ages and may move more often, an ambivalent relationship with one's accumulations grows. There can be a growing feeling that one is prisoner of one's stuff. But at the same time that it takes more energy and money to keep them up, things are also hard to part from. Identity is involved.

As one gets older the pile of things one has accumulated in a lifetime begins to morph. Reduction is setting in. Greater freedom lies with having less stuff. One is no longer so interested in spending time and energy on what was important in the past. Stuff soon feels like an obstacle. A new identity is emerging.

The process of paring down is reduction. Dreams and ambitions weigh heavy upon one. Becoming more true to oneself means handling each item and deciding where it fits in one's present life. This will mean less stuff and will become a familiar pattern to those who are willing to go through the sweet agony of surrendering.

Reduction alters the course of a life. It provides the circumstances of loss (or letting go) that arouses in us a creative response. There is a strange symmetry that reduction reveals; the more one becomes their unique self, the more one finds the unique service one has to render. In essence, one is reduced into place. Remember, this isn't just a human endeavor, this move is a far more complex maneuver than that. This is Nature, the life of the Universe, shaping us into, a fit that works for all. It is, from my viewpoint, evolution at work.

Reduction does diminish us. It fulfills the inevitable decline that is built into nature. And it is much more benign than that for it also provides a wind under one's wings, a natural clarifying force that enables one to ripen, to become the full essence of one's unique-ness, to be free like never before, to know one's relationship within all being. Oddly, diminishment of this sort brings happiness and a sense of lightening up, being less encumbered. The phenomenon of the paradox of reduction is not easy to convey.

Verification is underway in the life we have been given. It isn't there because of our efforts. It is there because Life intends something with us. Reduction doesn't remove all the questions, but it does point us toward the ones that really matter. The latter part of human life, the part that is dominated by diminishment and a lot of prejudice, is ac-tually a favor to us. Elderhood provides an opportunity that few of us are currently capable of grasping. The chance to become ourselves fully is real, and we are capable of serving just as we are. Elderhood is a ripening time!

Reduction also brings grief. This isn't one of the most popular attri-butes of being human. No one seems to want a life that is filled with grief. Reduction, however, gives grief a new meaning. Oh, there is still loss. Life shrinks, becoming something that is surely passing. It hurts to know that everything, including everyone, is passing, going into the inscrutable darkness.

Reduction makes this movement irrefutable. Death, the ultimate reduction, waits. The fact that death takes place offers a paradoxical understanding of the opportunity that Life actually is. There is something miraculous in everything that is passing so quickly. Impermanence reveals the preciousness of the moments we have. Grief is linked to praise. Each of them, grief and praise, are different facets of the same emotional reaction. These feelings arise when the whole specter of Life is apprehended.

Grief is the feeling of meaningful connection. It comes out when we humans feel that we have lost something important. Praise comes out when we feel that we are in the presence of something equally important. They each express a facet of the incredible gift that Life delivers. Sometimes the valued passes, and sometimes its value is around for just long enough to imbue us with meaning, awe, and a sense that life is worth living. Then, like everything, it passes. In so doing it creates this complex emotional experience.

There is grief and praise in letting go, voluntary or not. The field of connection is getting smaller, meaning it is concentrating in fewer and fewer relationships. Only those that are truly salient to the integrative process are left. Time is running short; so is life energy. Now relationships are so important that even good ones cannot stand the cut. Life is concentrating on adding the finishing touches. Elegance, beauty, meaning, spiritual integrity, and deep connection are now at the forefront of a shrinking agenda. This is most poignant and awe-inspiring.

The burn of loss is paradoxically the recognition of gain. Grief hurts, but not like a life that is empty of significance. To live fully is to lose everything completely. Grief never feels good, but it feels full. It is a gift of Life that brings tears and gratitude. So, grief becomes more palpable in later life. It offers to those who can give it an exalted position in their lives a perception of the beauty and poignancy of existence. It infuses life with praise.

Grief then is a phenomenon of later life. It is a recognition of how complexly composed everything is. When this perception settles in, when it becomes a part of everyday life, then strangely it joins with the other benefits of old age, and becomes an exquisite form of happiness. This happiness is a hallmark ingredient of elder awareness.

Nature always prevails. An old person's life is challenging. Life isn't fooling around. This period is laden with the possibility of actualization. Life is positively humming with potential. But little of it is accessible without the real ordeals that accompany it. The reality of the moment is that age brings one to the place of reckoning. Life is up for review. Now, one is confronted by oneself, the choices one has made, the person one opted to be, the alignment between the values one has aspired to, and the values one has lived by. The long arguments within oneself are settling.

There is a huge need for forgiveness and compassion in this place. If one does not love oneself enough, then this phase in Life makes that pretty evident. Old age, the proximity of death, the ravages of reduction, bring about a self-confrontation that is difficult, essential, and extraordinarily human. This is a very poignant and sacred enterprise. Self-reckoning is not the end of the story. For some, it is the motive for a new story. But, for it to be any of that, one must be able to look at one's life honestly, with a will to forgive and some understanding of what it means to be human.

All of this reckoning and the acceptance it requires prepares one for a beautifully freeing awareness. One has never really been in control. Surrendering the notion of control, the obligation one feels, the sense that one has to make everything come out like one wishes, is such a relief. It is a challenging relief, however. Surrendering is a developmental achievement. It introduces a new more complicated awareness. The practice of letting go to what is, of meeting reality on its terms, means opening up, giving up the illusion of control, and being available like never before.

This is an elder achievement that comes about as a result of loss. It is one that generates a lot of ambivalence. The boundary between adulthood and adult expectations, and elderhood and elder awareness is dense with uncertainty. Surrendering is one of the attributes of this dawning new awareness that conflicts with adult sensibilities, but never-the-less reflects a new level of maturation.

Reduction contains within it the paradoxical power that releases the new freedoms that come with loss. Learning how important surrender is to the process of becoming less physically able, while becoming more *internally* capable, is an essential ingredient of elder awareness. This kind of learning, however, because it runs across the grain of expectations, takes time. The practice of surrendering possessions, beliefs, relationships, and outcomes, aids the growth of this awareness, and helps with the preparation for death.

So, surrendering isn't just a spiritual practice; it is an essential component of Life. As Life takes away from us what we had formerly relied on, it is equipping us for the next phase. This is a pattern that some old people begin to trust. In essence, that is why one defining feature of the elder is a reduced fear of death. Life speeds us along an arc that is not really of our choosing. The merely older person, mesmerized by the losses along the way and still caught by the societal notion of adulthood, misses what the elder experiences — that each stage is also full of new gains.

Surrendering always involves giving up the illusion of control, and giving control over to something larger that is much more likely to be influencing the outcome. The Universe, which has been around for 13.8 billion years (so our scientists tell us), has been underway, generating galaxies, black holes, pulsars, and incredibly, Life, for all that time. Something is going on — The Universe is behind a movement that is so much larger than our individual lives. It was going on before we came on the scene, and it will be going on long after we exit the scene.

But, what is going on, and how does it shape our lives? No one really knows. The answer to these questions resides in the darkness that separates, and animates, the various pieces of the Universe. Amazingly, we humans are included in this incredible, mysterious energy phenomenon.

The Universe appears to be expanding through us. Life is an expression of that incessant activity. It is the energy that operates through each of us. Strangely, the Universe, through the aegis of Life, brings us into being, shapes what we call our lives, and then does something mysterious with us.

We are forced to give way to that mystery, not because we want to, but because Life possesses us rather than we possess Life. The heart of surrender is giving way to what carries us. It is an act of facing reality and not pretending to be bigger than Life. It is freeing, humbling, reassuring, and integrative. Happiness follows. Loss accompanies gain. Surrendering, the voluntary opening to the movement of life, allows Life to be what it is, and a people to be who they are.

There is a heartrending climax that faces each of us. No matter what we do, or have done, our lives go into the darkness. Death is very democratic; it happens to everyone. There are many versions of what happens next. But no one really knows. Those who have had near-death experiences say it is nothing to be afraid of. And that may be so. But death still represents a significant change of states. And for most of us that change is inscrutable and silent.

The older one gets, the further one enters into the "dying zone." Death is omnipresent here. This is frightening. Images of pain, disability and of loneliness are hard to avoid. In a death phobic culture this generates dread. Growing older threatens one's life. The end is nearer and more undeniable than ever. Strangely, or perhaps not so strangely, the proximity of death provides the cold dash of reality that makes living more vivid and gratifying than ever. This, too, is one of the wondrous (and too often un-talked about) attributes of getting older.

Life and death are inextricably linked. You can't really have one without the other. The one empowers and makes the other meaningful. I learned this the hard way, through being held on the edge of death for a long time, becoming disabled, and coming back to life as a senior citizen. Death begins long before the end. As one grows older, if one is not blinded by the ambient fear that permeates our culture, this becomes obvious. The assumption that death is only a biological necessity, forced upon us inevitably by our animal nature, leaves so much out.

For me dying started long ago. I didn't know it at the time. I was so intent upon living that I didn't notice death's first intrusions. I'm older now, and can see things I couldn't see then. Life is what is happening as I am making other plans. Death is similar (constantly interrupting), and has been with me all along. I am just getting old and mature enough now to see it.

Returning to life as an older, disabled man has been a real education. Death seems to be a ubiquitous part of life. For me, the luminosity and uniqueness of each thing, especially us humans, gains a special preciousness by virtue of the fact that all of it is impermanent. Death subtracts a bunch of possibilities from my life and gives me some new, unexpected ones that I haven't yet learned to fully appreciate. Growing older has made this apparent. I didn't set out to know what I do now. I want to do my best at describing what I have learned. Death is teaching me/us how to live.

Reduction isn't always as dramatic and big as it is in some lives, but even the little disappointments carry with them a bit of death. Life twists and turns like it does because death is omnipresent, working to dispel illusion and to bring people more fully to Life. The boy or girl who went somewhere else, the career that ended prematurely, the loss of a marriage, health, or economic opportunity, is a death. The painful things that make us who we are, are filled with the ministrations of death. Transitions of all sorts are referred to as death/rebirth experiences. That is because Life is not what it is, without death.

Life and Death, I've found as I have grown older, are closely aligned, so closely they are paradoxically related, both occupying the same space on the continuum. The end is just the beginning, not once, but over and over again.

Death for elders is not something to be dreaded and feared, but something that brings home the true mystery of this existence. What is remarkable about the outlook of the aged is not that death changes Life, but that Life changes death. Death is an aspect of Life, and for the elders amongst us, proof that Creation proceeds through their being. They are up to something, not because they have decided to be, but because their existence makes it so.

Death eliminates the superfluous and reduces us to what really matters. In so doing it introduces us to real life, to ourselves, and if we are really lucky, to the world that exists beyond our standard perceptions.

As one admits the reality of death into life, life takes on another hue; it becomes something precious, more lively, and gratifying than ever. Cancer patients report this all the time. The prospect of death enlivens them, and many say being terminal is one of the best things that ever happened to them. Life becomes more lively through the transforming power of knowing it will be over. The journey becomes more arduous and correspondingly, more beautiful because it has an end. Death can be an enlivening favor, a chance to be here like never before. This ensures that life is lived, by those who accept the invitation of death, to the fullest.

A change eruption of major proportions resculpted my life, dragging me into a new life and awareness. Death, if it doesn't kill one, reworks one. I learned the hard way that a part of one can die, the life I know can be taken away, and that one can be the phoenix and rise again. One, on rising is not, however, the same. I died a little, and lived anew.

What happened to me is perhaps more dramatic and thorough than most people experience. Having no choice, I got to experience death, and the way it can recreate a life. Ageing is death remaking one, the slow way. It favors the old, ripening them, and turning them into something savory and wise.

Death harbors another attribute that is paradoxical. It strips away a lifetime of presumed accomplishment, and reveals the essence of one's life. Wisdom and true knowledge come from the winnowing that accompanies life review and reductions. This is one of the secrets death cannot help but keep. The truth of essentializing is only unveiled through experience. The slow death of *shedding reduces the body, but reveals the self*, the essential dimension of who one is. Our culture suffers from not knowing about this inevitability, and from not knowing the core of our humanity is revealed in the latter stages of life.

They say "there are only two things about life that are certain: death and taxes." Now, it appears, reduction is too. Reduction reveals that death has been attending life all along. It has been actively making aspects of being alive more meaningful and vivid. At the same moment that it has been reducing us, it has been awakening us to reality. Loss and gain. They are elemental factors in human existence.

Like other good paradoxes, pain is joined with joy, loss with gain. One, can't have one without the other — they are like night and day, sunshine and rain. Elder life is not easy, because so much becomes evident, while everything is passing. Elder life, though, is strangely rich; it is filled with awe and a kind of raw and vulnerable happiness. Enchantment with life descends upon those living long enough and fully enough. This is a poignant occurrence. Having to experience loss in order to live fully — that seems, on the face of it, like a recipe for depression. And for some of us it is.

There is a larger picture, though. It comes into view later. It takes some ripening to get to it. Life cures us, by putting us under pressure, heat, pain, loss, age and death. All too many of us think this is cruel, but instead, it's a favor. The elders amongst us know this elemental truth, maybe not in so many words, but in a hearty and vital way. They have lived it. They have become ripe because of it.

Chapter 4
THE SURPRISING NATURE OF ELDERHOOD

Evolution has cooked up a historical era like none humanity has ever seen before. Evolution is changing the way the game unfolds, asking us all to play in a different way toward different ends. The evolution of awareness promises to be disruptive and, in fact, already is.

Life is taking on a new shape. There is a newer, more developed phase of human life in town. Elders are emerging, and they bring with them strange new capabilities. Old age is becoming something else. Old people, in larger numbers than ever, are waking up to a new life. Life is becoming richer, healthier, longer, more complex, relational, and full of new possibilities. Ripening is occurring.

Elderhood creeps into our lives rather unexpectedly. Many of us know we are going to die, but few of us really know that we are likely to live far longer than we are prepared for. Later life is more than a summary; it is refreshment. Like a deep, cleansing rain, the air is alive with renewal and possibilities are budding.

This isn't what we've been led to expect, and what is so exciting about it, is that a new, as yet unsettled landscape has become visible. The world isn't what it seems. We had been led to believe otherwise by our culture. The maps are being redrawn! Elderhood, as the unexpected extra time, is full of more than the inevitable decline that our society predicts. It is its own time of possibilities.

There is a new form of wisdom emerging now. This isn't just traditional wisdom. It is the wisdom of "not knowing." The future beckons more uncertainly than ever. Elder wisdom, today more than ever, is composed of the capacity to relate, and particularly to relate to the unknown. The future is calling to us in new and unknown ways, and strangely it is the new old who are most adept at listening. Elderhood makes "not-knowing" wisdom available. It offers a chance to step towards the unknown future.

Early adult life for us humans is primarily viewed as the time when we establish ourselves. This period of life is governed by heroic effort. Going out into the world, searching for one's place, determining one's contribution, and making one's mark; these are the concerns of this time. Busy-ness and doing are the indicators of worthiness. This is a time governed by cultural practices and beliefs.

Maturing asks us for more than we expect. Being culturally unprepared for a time of ripening, is one of the reasons so many don't become more, and end up merely old and cast away. Ripening is undesired, arduous, and strangely unexpected. Denial sometimes runs the show.

Perhaps this is the greatest transition a human being can make, and until now this shift, enormous as it is, has been treated like a human deficiency rather than an incredible achievement. Humanity suffers from assumptions that do not accurately reflect the complexity and beauty of Nature's design. We are stardust-confused, and aching because our imagination hasn't matched what Nature intends.

The shift toward a vital elder life is a turn inward, toward the heart of our being. Within is the new home of the elder. Life during this phase involves an integration that goes beyond the concerns and lessons of a culture that is obsessed with doing. Now a time of being is up, and what lies within is the passport to a better and more meaningful life. One can prepare for this possibility by living as fully as possible, but it doesn't happen because we humans want it to.

Something else makes that selection. That is why I say this moment reveals evolution at work. Humanity is being transformed, not through our own efforts (though it would be good if we cooperated), but because Life isn't through with us yet. The longevity revolution, and the demographic surge of the ageing baby-boomers, has set up a situation that is just as surprising for human culture as it is for human individuals. The time of ripening is surprisingly here. The human family tree is bearing gray fruit.

This is a moment like none other. There is a big, painful loss here. The end of productivity, in commercial terms, ushers in a difficult transition. Logic gives way to paradox. Welcome to the through-the-looking-glass world where loss is accompanied by gain. Welcome to the surprising world, where Life and Mystery are side by side, not to be resolved or solved in any way, but to be lived fully. Aging comes to us despite our will. It isn't a product of spiritual practice, psychological sophistication, or religious fervor; it is an unexpected gift from Life. Through some kind of strange evolutionary justice, this gift unfolds into being, as we respond to Life.

Old age contains many surprises to go along with the losses that it introduces. These are some of the gains. They make life richer and more enjoyable. But more importantly, they give Life new meaning. These attributes of later life make clear that experience, especially life experience, has a value that goes way beyond monetary wealth. The later years deliver one to an era of Life where there is a synergy between the wants and needs of the individual, with the wants and needs of Life. This synergy is palpable and results in gratification.

By being beyond productivity (in societal terms) — beyond the rules, roles, and social expectations — one finds a new freedom. Old age, by stripping people of their places in society, has performed the magic of liberating them. The bind of responsibility that one former-ly felt, is replaced by a lighter and deeper sense. What has happened is that aging has taken one to a place that is simultaneously simpler and lighter, while being more complex and choiceful. Freedom comes with an unexpected unburdening of an old skin. This freedom is self-won. It is the product of taking advantage of the newfound choices that accompany aging.

Relationship in particular benefits from internal freedom. The new old relate from a different place. They are free to enjoy the unique-ness of others. They are not threatened by the differences others embody. The fact that they are intrigued by differences and are less prone to be emotionally reactive gives them a greater relation-al capacity. This turns out to be one of the primary assets of aging. The ability to be with others non-reactively allows relationships to deepen and expand. All of this increases the meaning and emotional connection available, adding to the potential meaning that relation-ships can bring.

One of the key developments of human life happens in old age. People become themselves. Internal freedom translates into authenticity. Elders possess their true selves. They become the person they have always known themselves to be. There is no longer a divide between who one is, in any outer context, and who one is inside, in one's most private realm.

This is why the metaphor of ripening is so apt and powerful to the newly released. Life as an authentic, self-regulating, autonomous being has its own self-determined rewards. This newfound status as an actualized being is a joy to experience, and the gratifying outcome of a lifetime of struggle. It is a moment where liberation turns into an unexpected justice.

One becomes the gift one is. A lifetime of struggle to be oneself, to be true to one's uniqueness, comes to an unexpected fruition. Not only is there a realization of becoming the gift one is, but there is an equally powerful realization that one exists to give this gift of self to others.

Old people who have achieved this kind of ripeness are our truest veterans. They should be honored. They have not only survived and converted many difficulties into assets, but they represent what is best in human nature — the fulfillment of Life.

Freedom and self-possession add up to an unpredictable form of happiness. Researchers are beginning to show that the decades after 50 provide more and more happiness. Why is this? There are as many explanations as there are researchers, but it all comes down to a significant change of life. These are the decades when Life ripens old people, and some become elders. They have escaped the siren call of culture and have become themselves. That means that they aren't defined by what their parents were like, what job they had, how much money they have, or how educated they are. They are the products of their own determining.

Their happiness is deeper than just becoming themselves. There is a sense of alignment with the bigger picture. In the paradoxical world of the elder, the happy life is one of engagement with what is. It is a kind of recognition of the miraculous nature of the mystery that attends Life. It is the activity of being, the depth of perception that notices wonder. The world is re-enchanted, becoming a place where the unexpected delivers, and the unexplained explains. Don't-know mind dominates. Happiness is simply the thrill of being present, right in the middle of so much magnificence.

One of the many reasons for happiness in later life is how relational capacities change. Not for everyone, but for those who are becoming old in a new way. Aging changes some of our capabilities. What I am going to describe here is one of the potentials that all humans possess. This potential, which comes with age, was missed by the abbreviated attention of the Human Potential Movement. And, for that reason, along with the other surprises of old age, most old people don't even know that they are benefiting from the arising of this new capacity.

Old people, and especially elders, are a lot less emotionally reactive. They are able to go into relational places that they simply couldn't handle before. This means a lot of things. But basically, it means that elders are less likely to use violence and are much more interested in differences than ever before.

This advance, when looked at through the cultural perspective, is almost otherworldly. The human animal has long been considered violent. History seems to prove that. But, here, in aging, is also evidence that humans contain within them a capacity to ripen into nonviolence, to actually face Life as it is. Emerging right now, is awareness that we as a species are not doomed by our animal nature. We are animals that don't need to be forever fighting each other. Ripening arouses another possibility.

Elders are much more capable of being intrigued by differences. Besides, what this means for human-to-human relationships, think what it means evolutionarily. The ability to be less reactive translates into a greater acceptance of differences, and a greater acceptance of The Great Mystery. Later life, for some, reintroduces learning through renewed relationship and reduced emotional reactivity.

Relating to differences with intrigue instead of fear opens reality. This gives us chances we don't even know about. The happiness that accompanies elder life has the potential to change human life; this is a major part of why it should be known. The elder years hold a possible positive future at a time when dystopia, the product of our cultural imaginations, is the future we feed our kids. The kids benefit when there is a wide-spread recognition that life gets better.

By virtue of their maturity, life experience, and greater relationship skills, elders tend to be more emotionally intelligent. They are capable of seeing the world in ways that are not common to the rest of us. Because they have cultivated a kind of inner sight, as their inner lives blossomed, they are capable of perceiving a world that is invisible, a feeling realm. What they see, which is not apparent, are the lines of connection that emotionally link one thing with another. They perceive the ties that bind, and are increasingly aware of how things are paradoxically related.

This paradoxical awareness accounts for their increasing interdependence. They have acquired a kind of sensory apparatus that enables them to be aware of how embedded they are in a larger tangle of connections. This awareness, which often starts out simple, grows very complex. For most elders it starts out as a kind of fantastic discovery, a desire to relate more closely with family, especially younger generations (like grandchildren). In some cases, this new connectedness progresses to all humanity, living things, and the Universe as a whole. They, elders, are capable of experiencing relationship with it all.

The awareness of "all my relations" that some indigenous people achieved is not a product of their culture (though that certainly aided it); it is a design element of Nature. Humans are intended to know their place as evolutionary development happens. It is an awareness, which evolves with age. Elders are evolution incarnate. They have achieved an awareness that is built in. It is a complicated awareness that takes a while to unfold.

Everyone slows down as they get older. For a few it is part of an incredible shift, a reduction of speed, that allows something else to take precedence. For these few, slowing down brings with it a greater emphasis on the moment. Oddly, the less productive world of slowing down becomes the *more* productive world of leisure, reflection, integration, effortlessness and self-building.

The timelessness of slowing down makes living something else, and this allows the miraculousness of Life to become more palpable. This change of pace brings the self closer to the surface, enabling one to feel the natural unfolding of eternity. The slowing of Life, reintroduces one to Life, and highlights the enormity of what is happening. This realization leads one deeper into gratitude and increases reverence and happiness.

Only an old person can adequately convey what is like to live with the awareness of completion. I am not talking about being at the end; instead I'm referring to fulfillment. Imagine becoming all that one is, or having a sense of fulfillment and impending completion. Life ages us, until we achieve ripeness. This is a well-roundedness that leaves one feeling full of the miracle of becoming. To those who know this bliss, there is no more striving, there is only the precious chance to enjoy what is.

There is a form of innocent awareness that comes with later life. It isn't the innocence of childhood, naïve to the basic lay of the land, social arrangement, existential meaning, or relationship context. No, unlike childhood's innocence, which is born of knowing nothing, elder innocence comes about because elders have vast experience, and have freed themselves from the clutches of cultural (or other, outside) thinking. Elder innocence is grown into. It comes from the hard-won freedom of having lived through the assumptions of others and gone beyond them. That is why an observer of elder development (Dr. Allan Chinen), describes it as "emancipated innocence." Elder innocence is experienced and infused with freedom.

This renewed innocence allows the elder to experience Life as it is. Elders are enchanted all over again, not in the way of experiencing everything naively, but in experiencing everything again for the first time. Elders participate in a form of play that has been around since forever, but has remained poorly grasped. They really like hanging out together. This isn't just old folks desperately hanging out — to maintain some kind of recognition, dignity and way of passing time.

In this case, elders are coming together and playfully melding their consciousness, growing a more fluid awareness, and integrating that awareness into a form of consciousness more suitable for the actual complexity of Life. This form of play mixes spontaneity, laughter, reminiscence, perspective, experience, fluidity, humility and wonder. It is also a form of play that fulfills the instincts of the old. It is full of the subtleties, nuances and capabilities that come with maturity.

It is this quality of play, a special capability of the mature mind, that is the real reason learning in elder community is so compelling. There is no other social phenomenon that so replicates this unique attribute of elder life. Elders come together to fully integrate the special awareness that is dawning in them. They need each other, not like those who are dependently incomplete, but like those who are so full they need others to help digest the richness, complexity, and wonder of Life. When elders find the way to play together, integration takes place.

The future and the past are brought together. It is the kind of integrative learning that restores humanity's trust in existence. Life takes on the complex and wondrous fullness that makes being alive such an important opportunity. The Universe ages, and elders add wisdom to the unfolding.

Chapter 5
THE NON-CONVENTIONAL ELDER

The old hold a very special place in the ecology of human culture. They are the caretakers of the past, the ones entrusted with stewardship of humanity's traditions. As such they have served us all by being repositories of known wisdom. They deserve respect for that service. A service they provide quite organically. But an interesting thing is happening. Some old people are going further, they are becoming something new, becoming harbingers of an unfolding future.

This is a dramatic age. The future is in doubt. Some of the old are waking up with new abilities and new awareness. This defies expectations, the presumptions that any substantial change in humanity's abilities, would first show up in the young. But here is an irony. The old, by virtue of an increased life expectancy, and greater numbers, are the young of our time.

This phenomenon has never been seen before. The latter years are new — they provide a change that has not been fully integrated yet. A new story is emerging. The drama of this age now includes the emergence of an elder population, which has never existed in this way before.

And what elders are now bringing to the table is both known and unknown. By virtue of their longer lives and their more complex realizations they are much more capable of hosting the wisdom of our species. They are good advocates for the sensibilities and consciousness that has defined what humanity has become.

But, there is more. By virtue of their lengthened life expectancy, good health, and life-experience, some of them are embodying a form of consciousness that is extremely rare and nonconventional. These few, are revealing human potentials, that offer us a chance to address the present, and the future, in entirely unique ways.

One gerontologist, a Swede, Lars Tornstam (see Annotated Bibliography), who upon first noting this development, called it gerotranscendence. By that he was referring to a form of consciousness that some old people achieved (without trying) that perceived and related to things in a unique way.

It appears that some old people have acquired a sense of perspective that goes beyond what is currently considered conventional. Non-conventional awareness comes to the human mind slowly. It is the product and integration of many life experiences. That is why it is more prone to appear in the thoughts and feelings of the old. Unlike most old people, all of whom have had many experiences, this unique form of consciousness is catalyzed by a rare combination of difficult life experience (like illness, war, economic hardship, loss, oppression, death, or near- death experiences) and adaptive response. By the latter I mean that these particular people have been through something so challenging that it threw them temporarily into a place beyond all forms of intervention and evoked from them a response that is new, adaptive, and unusual.

What is so unusual about nonconventional awareness is that it surpasses this point, building upon unknowing and paradox, reaching an outlook that resembles normal experience but transforms it.

Time
The moment expands and, for some old people, the past and the future occupy it. Some old folks have a temporal perspective that includes generations, evolutionary dilemmas, cosmic time, and a sense of what Life is up to. They may appear disoriented, but in fact are acutely aware of the big picture and how it is unfolding in a circular rather than linear fashion.

Self
The sense of self amongst the nonconventional is paradoxical, solid in some circumstances and fluid in others. They have some certainty about having a self of their own (being filled with choices of their own making), feeling fully self-defined, while paradoxically experiencing themselves as mysteriously and uncertainly defined by something bigger. They respect a "higher power" and have mystifyingly become part of it. They are more self-confrontive, altruistic, and ego-transcendent. They have taken the average old person's concern with integration further by focusing upon larger, more holistic contexts.

Mystery
These old folks have a healthy regard for the unknown and tend to revere mystery. They accept what they don't know and go further by actually placing a lot of trust in the unknown forces at play in their lives. They enjoy the process of discovery while actively practicing letting go. They tend to have a very nontraditional spiritual orientation. They don't fear death. In fact, they typically seem to be at peace with it.

Relationship
The nonconventional have a greater than usual capacity for, and interest in relationship. These old folks prefer intimacy to superficiality. They tend to only invest in relationships that provide them with real connection. They know themselves and are, therefore, more available. They are skillful in their interactions, interested in others, good listeners, more accepting, and make meaningful connections. They do not adhere to social categories such as class, race, religion, education, economic status, age, or ability.

Advice
Life has thrown these people many screwballs, and they know it. Therefore, they have learned and been humbled. They take not-knowing very seriously. They have been through enough, and have a high enough regard for themselves and mystery, that they no longer make recommendations. They are not compelled by standard moral concepts; instead, they trust that the "higher power" knows what it is doing. They experience that it operates in unknown ways. Thus, they are supportive, compassionate and nondirective.

Diversity
Because of greater self-awareness and improved relationship skills, they are generally more capable of interest in different perceptions of reality, and more receptive. They have an intrinsic desire to know more, to inquire into differences, and the paradoxical ability to handle a more complex, baffling, and ambiguous reality. Conflict over differences is much less likely with them.

Inner Life
The nonconventional have a very active and rich inner life. They have escaped the pull of cultural practices and assumptions. They are autonomous and are now living a life that is more governed from the inside-out rather than from the outside-in. They are actively aware that the state of their relationship within governs what is possible for them without.

Solitude
They have a much more positive attitude about spending time alone. For them, time alone provides the opportunity to inquire more thoroughly within. Alone time enables them to align their actions with their values, sense of self, and spiritual beliefs. Solitudinal time nourishes internal development, and enables these old folks to solidify their own sense of what matters.

Death
To the non-conventionally minded old person, death is not such a fearsome prospect. Intrigue with Life and the trust of mystery carries

over to personal death. These older people exhibit a healthy regard for grief and the rigors of letting go, but at the same time, are not especially afraid of the mysteries associated with death. For them, death is part of the larger flow of life.

Playfulness
Being beyond the pull of others and of culture, leaves them to organize themselves in response to the moment. There is an attitude of playfulness and creativity that becomes a hallmark of nonconventional awareness. The responses to all situations are characterized by an attitude of wonder, joy, and play. People with this kind of awareness find Life stimulating, miraculous, and interesting. There is a general sense that all aspects of Life offer a wonderful chance to engage, be creative, play and learn. This is a way of being that is rich with an attitude born of what Dr. Allen Chinen calls "emancipated innocence."

Individuals displaying all of the attributes of nonconventional awareness are rare. It is much more likely that some old people will have, or show, only some of these characteristics. The awareness described above is catalyzed by life circumstances, situations that are totally idiosyncratic.

The old today, by virtue of their numbers, longevity, experiences, and energy, are much better prepared to make a real difference in our social interactions. Some of them have gained a more interdependent perspective. Some elders have capabilities that can lead to humanity's broader awakening. How? By using their new relationship skills to help other generations know their own possibilities. And by choosing to show up, making their capacities and perspectives known, not through teaching but by being exemplars, showing themselves, and revealing what is possible.

Nonconventional awareness comes attached to a kind of consciousness that represents human potential. *Our species is a very different one, depending upon which age perspective one looks at.* Elders reveal a species that is less dependent upon cultural reference points, and much more capable of taking in the nature of Life as it is.

Non-conventionality reveals something else about human life that it is good to know. There is an old saying that has been applied to saints and other spiritually advanced people: that they are "in the world, but not of it." That is a very apt description of the elder who has achieved a nonconventional perspective.

The opportunity that the new old bring is momentous. A new voice is arising. Elder awareness isn't even complete, but its voice is already complete enough so that it reveals new possibilities. For instance, it makes clear that Life accompanies us, despite our species' negligent behavior. Life has grayed some fruit just for this moment. Aging, it turns out, is a form of ripening — a process of becoming viable seed. Old people reveal the on-going, juicy nature of Life. Life is creating new Life, and old folks, at least some of them, are already a part of this incredible, just-breaking phase of evolution.

Chapter 6
ELDER DEVELOPMENT

———

"Aging is not a process of inexorable decline, but a time for the progressive refinement of what is essential."
— CARL JUNG

Old age is an altered state. It is like taking a hallucinogen. The familiar takes on an unfamiliar, disorienting, and beautiful shape. Reality gains in liveliness. Formerly discrete things start to merge. The prevailing assumptions, the things one learned in the past, are not as reliable as they once were.

Old people are having their consciousness rearranged. This isn't a voluntary change. It is one comparable to gaining sex characteristics in puberty. Because this change is not recognized or voluntary, there is still a lot of confusion aroused by it. People resent what they cannot understand. The old feel like a crippling disease has overcome them; and, by and large, the young feel like the old are breaking down. This is only the appearance of things. As psychoanalyst R. D. Laing once said, "all breakdown isn't pathology, some of it is breakthrough." Old people are moving on, thanks to Life, to a new form of awareness.

It is worth repeating that all old people do not have the same experience. As I have stated elsewhere some old people, the majority, are merely older. The onset of a new, more emotional intelligence does not arise uniformly. Extensive factors ensure that only a minority of old folks are subject to this kind of overwhelming awareness.

An older person, oriented more from within than without, destined to become more unique, and growing into a more nonconventional perspective, is becoming less scientifically real as time passes. The passageway or initiatory ordeal that faces the maturing one is nothing less than a death and rebirth. It is a death to what was once considered real, and a re-birth to a new perception of reality.

Human development proceeds past childhood. It goes on through adulthood and, with these observations, on into elderhood. There seems to be a kind of logical progression. It goes like this: dependence, independence, interdependence. Human development seems to proceed from a strictly outside dependence to a more inside autonomy and on into a firmly inside awareness. This movement changes the meaning-making process, re-locating meaning from an outside awareness of others, through a more internal awareness of self, toward a greatly internal awareness of the energetic ties that connect.

Here are the unexpected tasks that occur with prolonged aging. These developments lead up to a most essential surprise — our presence in Life is not an accident. These tasks each seem unpredictable, even unlikely, becoming most probable in later life, and they make the process of becoming an elder something of a coming home to our species' true nature. With age the likelihood grows of:

- becoming more fully oneself,
- discovering how to best serve,
- aligning those two developments,
- and learning through community.

Nature endows each of us with the capacity to become ourselves, to find personal fulfillment in our old age. That is news, good news to the up-coming baby-boomers, those millions who are greying the world and who will have 20 to 40 years of life left to figure out how to age well. Life is not over. Instead, Life seems to be creating something new — a cadre (perhaps millions) of human beings that reveal to all of us what is possible. Life seems to be prevailing through transforming us into more complete beings.

Through some kind of numerical alchemy, each new level of awareness is less numerous than the previous one. Higher consciousness, as it grows, becomes rarer and rarer. New awareness appears in small minorities. As few as 5 to 7 out of 100 old people become elders (in the sense I am using the word), and only one or two in every hundred elders become non-conventionally aware. This fact is what's happening. Nature is retooling human life. Some of the old are becoming the new.

The old are just swollen with the desire to give, with an impulse to serve, that finds no obvious outlet in our youth-oriented culture. The life experience, learning, and perspective of the old are pretty much ignored now. This is a wasted resource, the neglect of which extracts a toll on elders, families, culture and our species' future.
As one grows older, life changes, often in very unpredictable ways. These changes precipitate new awareness. Surviving difficult challenge sensitizes one to the value of challenge, and to the rigors of responding. This has a humanizing effect.

Add to this, the maturing process elders undergo — lining up their desire to be themselves with their burgeoning desire to serve — and you have a recipe for growing empathy. This process of alignment happens as folks become older and the desire to give grows. The stronger the feeling of self-possession the more unique becomes the contribution. As these two elements of advancing age increase, the more they come into alignment, the more one experiences altruistic impulses.

Alignment like this, isn't available to everyone. It is part of our species' potential, but because we haven't really recognized the potential that resides in elder development, it isn't widely actualized. The amazing thing is, that even with the neglect and prejudice that is heaped on the elderly, some achieve it anyway.

Growing older is just that: growing. Elders are learning at an accelerating pace —that learning is self-directed, choice-full, tuition-free, and entirely experiential. In the process, elders are learning how to best be themselves. They are learning how to give the truest gift they have to give to others (and this incredible human experiment).

To have the opportunity to go back to learning completely on our own terms, is a big surprise. In so many ways elders are being tested— not by teachers or professional bodies — but by Life. And the testing is bringing out aspects of nature that are unknow. At last, elders are getting to familiarize themselves with their own deeper selves. No one ever anticipated that aging could stimulate this kind of growth.

Nor would people have anticipated how much community would mean. It is a surprise that people feel more capable of relating than they ever have. It is a further surprise when a social connection, particularly with a community of peers, sustains one so much. When learning, the feeding of an elder's curious mind is combined with community; the feeding of one's desire for meaningful connection, and this combination brings about transformative learning.

There is so much we don't know about ourselves. Human beings need to be in community with others to know ourselves better, to know others better, and to discover what being human is all about.

When old folks awaken to the fact that they hold some of the keys to the future, then something miraculous starts to happen. A new sense of dignity begins to emerge. The future is not just in the hands of, or a sole concern of the young. When the old contribute, then fresh possibilities exist for everyone. The more empowered they are, the more they contribute. This is the real antidote to the problem of the future of social security — connections made valuable, and meaningful, by real, caring interactions.

This has been quite a development. No one could have predicted it — or made it happen— but elderly people are capable of it. Fabulous elders thrive in this kind of nutritious environment — where mutual feeding takes place.

The process of discovering how to create community liberates social capacity. Elder potential is best emancipated by the use of elder capacities, capacities that remain unknown until they are unleashed. This is the great empowering secret of elder community. It is a great surprise to discover late in life, that the skills needed to fulfill one's self lie within, awaiting oneself and others to activate them. Together in community, elders have discovered that the adventure of being human, even an older human, is so much richer, when others share it. This learning has brought home the importance of community to growth and development.

These tasks represent a maturation process. Wisdom is a product of that maturity. Currently, we are in a society that doesn't value or recognize maturity. Our obsession with staying young, and with youth culture, reveals how little concern there is for growing up. This rebounds against the elderly and especially elders.

Elder development involves the hard and ultimately painful task of being true to oneself. Elders serve best, by holding on to themselves, showing up, and exemplifying an alternative way of being. Compassion, understanding, stolidness, trust in the whole, and connection, are the elements they embody and exemplify.

When a human individual graduates to becoming of service to the whole, to becoming an instrument of evolution, then that individual has learned where personal development, and the growth of the whole intersect. That is a spiritual development.

The phenomenon of aging into an elder is a complex mix of human development, yearning to serve, growing meaning, and the ministrations of Life. I think that scientific tools are just not subtle enough to capture the fully nuanced beauty of this form of transition. It allows one the chance to become something else.

What passes for wisdom today is so pedestrian. Mystery has been leached from it. This is the effect of believing that science and education address everything, and that soon all that is unknown will be known. Technology seems to imply that all things will one day be under control. It is as if evolution isn't happening, and as if the Universe isn't expanding.

Old age brings this awareness back again. There is something about surviving a near miss, an actual uncertainty-rearing hardship, which rekindles wonder, placing one appropriately, humbling one, and re-enchanting the world. Living near death, being aware of the fragility of existence, seems to generate a different sense of perspective. In old age the possibility of relating deeply and humbly enough to access this form of wisdom is greater than at any other point in life.

The journey of a lifetime leads to some possibilities that have never existed before. The old are a kind of advance guard. Some of them are showing the rest of us what is possible. The emergence of this development has deep implications for us as a culture. The fact that some old folks age into it, shows that it is a naturally occurring part of our species' potential. We need to know that. Within all of us there resides the capacity to see the greater picture of reality. The scope of the Cosmos lies within us. Aging enhances the chances that this kind of awareness be made more available.

Chapter 7
INTEGRATION

The last phase of life has to do with putting all of one's life into a sensible arrangement. This is an interesting process. It's completely idiosyncratic. Integration isn't an intentional human endeavor. It goes on anyway. People often come to the end of their lives wondering what it was all about. Integration can help make sense of one's existence. It may or may not close the circle. Integrative ripening is happening despite the assumptions that we as cultural beings or as individuals bring to the matter.

Nature, it seems, has seen fit to help individuals of this species come to the end of their line as fully human as possible. This move manifests in a variety of ways. This is what makes it so hard to identify. Memory, motivation, relationship, physical aging characteristics, meaning-making, reminiscences, spiritual and religious desire, and even altruistic impulses can be expressions of this unitive force. Perhaps this is some late-breaking instinct, but whatever it is, it aids us. It provides support for actualizing, and making use of our existence.

A natural design element of later life is the integrative force. Nature helps us be all that we can be. This help defies our assumptions. Nature is not interested in competing with us to provoke variation. Evolution is backing us, helping us fit into the larger picture better. Later life is a time when this force serves us.

Nature ripens us. It is busy within us — without our agreement — and until now, without our knowledge. We are more valuable to evolution than we think. Our lives are not simply our own. The integrative force is the expression of the Universe cohering. It operates in all our lives because it is operating throughout Life. We are simply beneficiaries.

There is a continuum of connection that runs through the personal experiences of each of us humans, right on through to what is going on at the largest levels of the Universe. Integration isn't just about becoming all one can be. Integration means lining up several dimensions of experience. It involves connecting all the dots.

Fortunately, some of those dots become more explicit in later life. The act of reminiscing about foregone experiences might just be a reclaiming, or re-understanding, something important. Maybe a quality of life, a relationship possibility, or a disappointment, bring home an aspect of loving. The poignancy of long-term memory is breathtaking. When these-kind-of-memories get translated into meaning, this alters one's regard for Life, and then something gets stirred at a larger level. Living informs the ongoing process of Creation.

Summing up, coming-to-a-conclusion, having one's own guess about the purpose for one's life, serves the ongoing pursuit of Life, and makes the personal dimension of existence clearer. This is the opportunity that resides at the end of the trail. It represents the greatest highlight — when one gets to know the magnificence of living.

Integration in a human life is a complex phenomenon. There are certain characteristics of this process. They reveal a lot about the state of one's life. There is almost nothing external that can be dependably relied upon to evaluate the elder. It is the quality of one's inner life that differentiates individuals.

Here are the hallmarks of a well-integrated life. These are the indicators that reveal balance. No one person is likely to have fully developed each of these dimensions, but the old one who is truly an elder has all of them fully underway. The hallmarks are;

- freedom

- integrity

- happiness

Freedom
The latter part of life, is the time old people are most likely to become themselves. It is then that they are developing a much stronger capacity to live from the inside out. That means that they are motivated much more by intrinsic (inner) drives than extrinsic (outer) ones. They are living much more on their own terms. They are not governed nearly as much, if at all, by a desire to be socially acceptable. In essence this time of life is when they are much more likely to feel its time to be authentic. It's like one 86-year-old woman said to me, "It's now or never."

It is a strange twist of fate, when an old one realizes that freedom isn't, by itself, enough. This realization makes a more-full form of integration likely. It brings out despair and disappointment. One has to have achieved a sense of being fairly free, to even get this kind of awareness. Happiness about self-possession turns into uncertainty. Life is even more complex than becoming unique. Freedom, the thing many struggle all their lives for, isn't enough. Liberating and being oneself, is not the end of the story. If elders were not experiencing the onset of a more paradoxical awareness, this achievement (of realizing there is more development they can do) would threaten them; but instead it just motivates them toward deeper and broader aspirations.

Integrity
Like freedom amongst elders, there is a natural desire to live life based on the coherence of one's self-selected values. Self-respect depends upon the self-evaluation one gives oneself. Self-love demands adherence. Elders are pinned down by the choices they have made, and resolute about applying the creativity of their own values to whatever may come.

This attribute is the heart of integrity. However, it is a deceptive thing. Because, by itself even integrity suffers when it isn't accompanied by freedom and happiness.

The desire to live a life of integrity can become rigid. Integrity can seem like a justification. People forget all about surrender and letting go. They become so solid that they are unable to bend. When this happens, then integrity isn't enough to assist integration. An old one like this, is likely to be troublesome and non-relational. Isolation haunts the one who places too much emphasis upon integrity. Things look different with paradoxical awareness. Integrity can become its opposite.

Happiness
The natural exuberance of Life comes through some elders. They feel joy just from being alive. With integrity and freedom enough, this joy can go so far as to acknowledge the sorrow in the world. Life becomes bittersweet. The old person can see the horrors of the world paradoxically, right beside the miraculous nature of things. This is truly a happiness born of the realization of wholeness, of the Oneness that underlies all things. To be a part of that wholeness, and to be authentically oneself — that is beyond any kind of undoing.

But happiness, too, can be not enough. Too much of an emphasis upon happiness can be a way of bypassing the real pathos that comes with Life. There can be an over-reliance on happiness, which can lead to a more pleasant form of rigidity, but a form of rigidity never-the-less. Happiness can be denial. Life is beautiful. It has a quality that is very stirring. And yet, part of that quality is poignant and some-times rough. This, too, is an essential aspect of the whole. Integration doesn't stop here — but it does visit —and elderhood means going with it.

The new elder carries a momentous responsibility. This responsibil-ity comes with ripeness. It is time to put childish things down. Elder-hood, the rising of the third moon, is fateful. It offers a useful pinnacle for us to climb, making of this advance of Life a more well-rounded starting place toward aligning human consciousness with the purposes of Life.

The Universe is not literally teetering upon our choices, but something is happening. The increasing numbers of the old portend an opportunity. The wave-front of the silver tsunami is just before us. This is a time of change, one that offers us, as a species, something needed — the opportunity to grow up and evolve by becoming more. This is an opportunity for humanity to age well.

Chapter 8
ELDER PLAY

---

*"Playing together is perhaps the most profound way
of communicating unconditional love."*
— ANDREW GREELEY

As people age, their way of perceiving the world changes. Humorists know this. Stand-up comedians customize their material based on their perception of the make-up of their audience. Age is one of the factors considered. Why? Because there is some recognition that age changes the funny bone. Play is similar. What is compelling, engrossing, and fun changes as we age, as does the ability to interact, and the perception of what is salient and meaningful. Life is fun in different ways.

Good humor is a universal component of play, and a sense of good humor also ages, becoming more complex, nuanced, and sensitive. The advantages of a long, much experienced, life full of paradox, reversals, and wonder, and makes elder play harder to grasp. Older people don't only play differently from younger folks, they value the whole of life differently. Old people, especially elders, carry around altered brains, changed consciousness, paradoxical awareness, and a familiarity with death that deepens and further democratizes their play, making of it an exquisite way to integrate all that they are experiencing.

Elder play happens spontaneously, and for its own sake. It isn't really Bingo, Bridge, or Golf. All of those games could be an invitation to play; it could happen there, but real elder play happens anywhere at any time. It is an expression of an attitude that goes beyond the forms of the moment, and often punctuates what's happening with delight and mischievousness. Elder play is exuberant, and enthusiastic about the mysteriousness of life.

So, what is it about elder play that warrants attention? Why is it important? Because the opportunities for this unique form of interactive creativity are so limited by prejudice, misunderstanding, and an overly busy lifestyle that the special perspective old age offers, is frequently lost. This, hurts elders a lot, denying them the chance to be all they can be. It also hurts everyone else. Social reality suffers, when the broader perspectives of elders are ignored. Elder play is a fundamental location for this expanded perception.

Old people are typically well versed in the ups and downs of life. A primary benefit of all of this experience, is that some people realize, that how they respond to the adventures and uncertainties of Life, makes a difference in how they experience Life. As a result, they often cultivate a more playful way of responding to what Life throws at them. They can be serious, and often are, but at the same time, they can meet what Life serves up, with an attitude of openness, anticipation, wonder, and playfulness. They know that their existence is defined, in part, by their willingness to enjoy the Life they have. This attitude reflects awareness that Life is much more than our culture presumes. After a long exposure to Life, a small number of old people, whom I call elders, come to the place in themselves where they feel a desire to cooperate with Life.

This attitude of playfulness isn't just a new elder development. All age groups have been privy to the kind of awareness, that breeds this tremendously adaptive response to Life. As one grows more present within the moment, then those possibilities become more palpable. Old people, by virtue of their short-term memory changes, are thrust into the moment. When this awareness is combined with the attitude of playfulness, then the moment becomes a rich opportunity to experience more of the nuances and beauty of Life.

This is an attitude, that is born out of an ability to extend oneself creatively into any situation. The attitude of playfulness is like the acceptance of a good improviser. "Yes," is the keyword that precedes the art of improvisation. So too, the playful person says "yes" to Life. This "yes" comes from within, and is lived out in all circumstances.

Elders, through their playful attitude, are actively merging the personal with the collective. They are taking what Life gives them, and finding ways of transforming their experience into a form of nourishment. This is not merely an adaptation to the challenges of existence; it is a way of converting those experiences into a rich loam for others. When an old person adopts and cultivates an attitude of playfulness, they are re-enchanting the world, and demonstrating the connective power that resides in it. This has an impact on consciousness, and might very well change the world we live in. Evolution is shaking the tree, and grey fruit is playfully falling out.

I'm going to rely on the expertise of Dr. Peter Gray. He is a professor emeritus from Boston College and an evolutionary psychologist who has studied play. His observations bring out some of the most salient attributes of play, and reveal how this activity has such a profound impact upon determining what is socially achievable. Through his eyes we can see something of what elder play holds for us all.

One of the primary characteristics of good play is freedom. An axiom of play theory underscores this point, "One cannot play if one has to." To play one must be free enough so that, as Peter Gray says, one can "quit." It is the ultimate democratic impulse that keeps play free, not only by virtue of completely autonomous participation, but play must be free of objectives. Play is paradoxical. It provides many benefits, but only freely provides them if they are not sought through the liberating nature of play. Play must be free and susceptible to change, not to an imposed agenda — even of the most well-meaning sort — to really be play.

Elders, because they are so self-possessed, and have gained the mature capacity of being true to themselves, are naturally free. This makes play very attractive to them. It is a self-chosen way of exploring and developing creative means for responding. Play is an activity. It is a means of engagement. What makes play so unique is that it isn't interested in the outcome, as it is in creating new and different ways of engaging. The more creative one's engagement is the more satisfying the play.

Its voluntary nature makes it a powerful vehicle for all kinds of free associations, behaviors, and trials. Socially, playing together while maintaining freedom, encourages participants to learn how to please themselves while pleasing others. Self-motivation has a way of becoming larger than the skin-encapsulated self, because play naturally calls out of us the larger dimensions of freedom.

"Play is a freely-chosen activity, but it is not a free-form activity." Play contains a wonderful paradox, one which prompts the kind of integrative development that is the hallmark of old age. The desire to play is so strong that it motivates the ones who play to use themselves well within the parameters (or rules and structure) of play. Thus, play evokes self-knowledge and self-discipline.

The structure of play is like the structure of any moment in Life. By playing within that structure, that is, freely engaging with what is, then one finds an opportunity to discover and express a freely chosen response, which comes out of the self.

Play contains yet another paradox that empowers it: the real is imaginative and the imaginative is real. Play is removed from the world, yet is deeply of the world. From this paradoxical formulation, it is easy to see that play is a natural expression for the ones who are in the world but no longer of it (nonconventional elders). The imaginative dimension of play allows the world to expand. Make-believe becomes make-it-so.

Play provides an opportunity to examine a scenario, and to find a way of responding to it, that is propitious. Such a response is consistent with elder responsibilities and elder freedom. Remember elder life is lived with an expanded sense of self, which makes playing an excellent way of exploring the mysteries of expansion. This activity, conducted in this way, is thoroughly aligned with evolution.

"Because play involves conscious control of one's behavior, with attention to process and rules, it requires an active, alert mind." The ballast of a well-developed self, is actually what allows for relaxation, and the recognition of the saliency to self, is what sharpens attention. Relaxation and alertness are not qualities of mind alone; they are qualities of development.

Presence is an elder strength. And that includes presence of mind. When a circle of elders concentrate on some shared issue, they travel together into a state of mind that is full of inquiry, good humor, and attention. There is a tendency to notice the obvious, and then to go further, and observe the overlooked. All the while there is delight, poignancy, grief, and wonder. A native intelligence, a shared intelligence that arises out of the presence of those present, which looks into differences, stimulates the mind and enlarges perception.

Play, as an elder, is very different from play as a child. The elder looks out into a world that is as enchanted, as the one the child is privy to, but the elder has endured a period where the magic seemed to have disappeared. The return to the world of miracles is a journey that no child has experienced, and a young one knows little of the long-life journey that makes such awareness possible again. The journey from childhood wonder to elder awe, is not a short one, and has no usual features, but it does have regular stops, and these include: an extension of the continuum of awareness, an increasing integration, a celebration of Life, and a desire to share the miracles of Life.

The integrative force seems stronger in some lives. Play for some elders is a necessity, like food. It nourishes something living within. Elder play is suffused with a mature desire to share the miraculousness of Life. Play, seems to some, to be a more interactive and fun form of prayer. It isn't the form of prayer that is asking for anything; play is, for some elders, praise for what is.

The play of the elder commonly manifests as a spontaneous expression of the moment. Elders experience the moment differently; they are privy to a more expanded experience of the now, which makes them seem preoccupied and inattentive. Some of elder attention goes into the nooks and crannies of the moment. They are noticing the nuances, experiencing a broader movement implicit in the now.

Thus, they have a facility with the moment that comes out in their humor. This kind of playfulness is infectious. It builds community — a community of fun. People pick up this tendency and soon this form of playfulness becomes a playful way of connecting with each other.

You have heard about how growing old generates a "second childhood." Well, there is some truth to that perception. There is one big exception to this take, though. Elders <u>progress</u> into a new form of innocence, <u>instead of regressing</u>, which is the present popular assumption. The playful attitude that characterizes elder awareness, is born from experience, not the loss of awareness. Elder playfulness is a hallmark of a truly mature person.

There is a form of innocent awareness that comes with later life. Unlike childhood's innocence, elder innocence comes about because elders have vast experience and have freed themselves from the clutches of cultural or other outside thinking. Elder innocence is grown into; it comes from the hard-won freedom of having lived through the assumptions of others and gone beyond them. That is why an observer of elder development, Dr. Allan Chinen, describes it as "emancipated innocence." Elder innocence is experienced, and infused with freedom.

This new, free innocence allows another interactive phenomenon, that is very poorly understood. Elders participate in a form of play that has been around since forever, but has remained poorly grasped. They really like *hanging out* together. This isn't just old folks desperately hanging out, to maintain some kind of recognition, dignity, or way of passing time. This is actually real play, the paradoxical interactive pursuit of a larger awareness.

Elders are coming together, and playfully melding their states of consciousness, growing a more fluid awareness, and integrating that awareness into a form of consciousness, more suitable for the actual complexity of Life. And they do it, through simply interacting about most anything. This is a kind of play that is unselfconscious. In fact, many old folks are not even aware that they are playing as they interact. Everything happens too naturally to be anything, and that is exactly what makes it play. This form of play mixes spontaneity, laughter, reminiscence, perspective, experience, fluidity, humility, and wonder. It is also a form of play that fulfills the values of the old. It is full of the subtleties, nuances, capabilities, and the happy humor that come with maturity.

Elders come together to fully integrate the special awareness that is dawning in them. They play and discover themselves together. They need each other, not like those who are dependently incomplete, but like those who are so full they need others to help digest the richness, complexity, and wonder of Life. When elders find the way to play together, integration takes place. There is a kind of whole-organism, experiential learning possible in old age that is essential to our species' wellbeing.

There seems to be some instinctive elements to learning, that ensure that we, as social animals, pass along our social/cultural nature. Later life is when the big picture becomes more evident. It is when humans are more amenable to encountering reality as it is. These aspects of integrative learning provide a better grounding for cultural endeavors.

Human aging combined with historical longevity, has evolutionary implications. Old folks, particularly the rare elder, are evolution at work. The new elder is a harbinger. Greater maturity is disruptive — but not like the evolutionary cul-de-sac of immaturity. The future is beckoning to us, through elder awareness.

Chapter 9
EVOLUTION AND RIPENING

———

Evolution is bringing to us a new, more complex awareness, an unexpected sense of maturity. Things are not what they used to be. People don't realize that evolution is happening right now. It is changing the playing field, as it always has. Changing it this time, in a most unusual way — a way that defies our species' expectations. To give the experiment of Life a better chance, evolution is doing something that is not intuitively obvious. It is remaking the old into the new.

By adding life expectancy, and by increasing the numbers of people over the age of 65, social reality is changing. The old are new. They soon will be a significant percentage of our population. Maturity is taking on new proportions. Human awareness and behavior is developing a new range.

This new maturity may, or may not, be enough to save us from ourselves. The hole we have been digging is deep. Another further, historical development is that humanity is living with the realization that we humans have the wherewithal to put an end to ourselves, and all complex life on our planet. We now know, like never before, that we can generate collapse!

The generations that have come after the first nuclear bomb are living in a world that is different from what any of our ancestors knew. Some of those who are reaching elderhood, now are the first to live their entire lives under the shadow of human-generated anni- hilation. Collapse is now a possibility! Conditions have changed. This awareness has altered the backdrop of modern life. Our existential awareness has been added to by the deepening realization of our en- vironmental impact. We, especially those becoming elders now, are being affected.

Life pushes us into the future. This movement isn't always easy or elegant. Evolution expands consciousness by never covering the same ground twice. Like the spiral, Life pushes the movement of evo- lution through ever-expanding stages. This movement shows that Evolution, following a spiral design, keeps the past embedded within it, while reaching for a larger, more expansive future.

Evolution reaches for a new perspective while including and going beyond the old. This accounts for familiarity and the sensation of a recurring cycle, while it explains the acquisition of something new to be integrated. Life is constantly playing through our lives, disturbing us, and delivering us to new challenges that require new ways of op- erating. The role Life plays in shaping us is made even more obvious as we age. Life has its way with all of us, and as it does, we spiral into what evolution intends.

While no one can predict what the future may hold, I think it fair to say that life-extension and the surge in the numbers of old folks, suggests that an important change is already underway. To grow, we have to abandon our own achievements. We have to enter a larger, more complex realm in order to actualize the potentials inherent in us. The pattern is loss and gain. To be alive, to thrive and to grow, involves constantly going through the process of surrendering the past, in favor of meeting the unknown and unguaranteed future.

The losses of life are organic. They are not a tragedy. Yes, they hurt. But, they are part of a larger movement. One that is paradoxical. Evo- lution, and its proxy Life, moves from one stage to another. The com- bination of loss and gain occurs along the way.

Human life is a rollercoaster ride, filled with ups and downs. The ups are thrilling, the downs, destabilizing, painful, and fraught with uncertainty. They are all paradoxically related. Old folks, most notably elders, know this pattern, and are less likely to judge any portion of it. For this reason, elders are less emotionally reactive, and more likely to be more objective about the ups and downs.

Some old people have lived long and hard enough to know this. They can see the connection between what they have been through, and the larger patterns of Life. Their lives reflect the way Life moves through us. Therefore, they have some understanding of the thrust of Life, and how it mirrors the processes of evolution. They represent a chance for us as a species to make an adjustment, to align ourselves, and our lives with the larger patterns of Life.

Human maturity is difficult because it is something so awesome and paradoxical — complex and simple, and yet more accurate and demanding. And as we are seeing here, it is an expansion. The arc of evolution is growing again, taking us beyond ourselves.

Elderhood is itself a form of initiation. It is an unusual one, not a man-made time of duress, made to deliver one to a new level. Instead, it is a Life-made immersion in the hardships of existence, designed to deliver one to the fullness of being human — it is an actual ripening, meant to bring out the uniqueness of each one of us.

And, like our bodies, it is more complex than our understanding. Our scientific acumen is not as extensive and formidable as our natural inheritance. Life has done a good job of providing us with capacities beyond our current state of knowledge. Growing, as it turns out, isn't just a voluntary effort. Life exceeds our expectations. In this case, growing us, making us an older, more mature, and capable animal.

This is a transformation that is way beyond our expectations. Life is modifying us, changing the playing field, adding to our nature, and extending us by clarifying our possibilities. We are being taken beyond ourselves.

Life's initiation strips down the superficial, and lets the superfluous go, in favor of the essential. Loss is painful, uncertain, and humbling. So, sometimes, is gain. This initiation is no picnic. It is an advanced adult activity. The rigors that come with this stage of life, provide the perspective and maturity, which account for wisdom. Life is the wellspring of this fresh insight. Without initiating hardships, the sensibilities that uplift us, would not be available. These initiating hardships are Life's way of growing us.

It is as if Life is creating a way for human beings to go beyond the patent assurances of culture to a fresh awareness, less contaminated by past assumptions. It seems elders are reaching a kind of escape velocity where they may no longer be bound by the gravitational pull of mass mind. Cultural inheritance is giving way to natural inheritance. In this new orbit not-knowing is far more useful — it is a more creative way of grasping the reality of the moment than the knowledge of the past.

Elder perception is coming from the awareness that more knowledge, reveals more of what one does not know. This realization sets one free from the binding weight of convention. This can be, for most, a terrifying and fruitful liberation. It opens the mind, and creates a new mode of perception.

The unique perspective of elder awareness, by virtue of new social capabilities, can become a synergetic consciousness. This new collective awareness is capable of a form of wisdom much larger, more nuanced, and spontaneous than any past knowing. Paradoxical thinking ensures this kind of awareness, as it is a product of both/and thinking instead of either/or, so it includes the knowledge of the past, without privileging it.

What interests me about the nature of this moment of evolution, is that the individual and collective are all evolving at once. This is a thoroughgoing change. Elder awareness is breaking out, wherever humans are living longer. As a species-wide change it isn't uniform, and doesn't alter everyone, but this elder-making initiation changes the repertoire of the species, transforming its range of options.

The new elder isn't different, and valuable, because of more knowledge; rather, an elder's value comes from *who* they are. They have integrated what Life confronts us all with. They have had many experiences that cannot be put in a textbook, or even an account of elder similarities. Living has made them unique and, paradoxically, a part of an overall movement that is Life growing itself.

Life has engineered a change, altering the consciousness of an entire species by changing the awareness of some of its oldest members. This isn't just a change in our knowledge base. We know enough to live better, to make living more sustainable. Life is catalyzing a change in our species' character, an added depth.

Thanks to some of our most aged ones, our species has a chance it didn't have before. We, as a species, have entered an historical era where, for the first time, we know our species death is possible. We now have to live with the backdrop of self-annihilation. We know, like never before, that we hold our own fate in our hands. Like it or not, deny it or not, the truth is that awareness of the end, species' death, is everywhere. It resides in the number of apocalyptic visions we harbor, and in the widespread social (and cultural) distrust that haunts us. Where are the images of a future worth having? Death of all humanity is a possibility that cannot be ignored.

This is where the elder experience with death and loss could be particularly helpful. Many elders have used awareness of the presence and inevitability of death to enliven their remaining days.

The wheel of fate is spinning. No one knows for certain what is going to happen. The moment is deeply uncertain. The human experiment teeters on how we handle this opportunity. Maybe the scientists are right, and it's already too late to save the human experiment. That does not preclude humankind from living more fully, possibly actualizing more of our potential. It just might be that our finest hour is our last.

I am not presuming this is the end. I think, instead, it is a beginning. But I have lived long, and uncertainly enough, to know that if the moment isn't as full of uncertainty as it is, it wouldn't contain as much potential as it does. It is up to us, and our partner, Life, to make of this moment what it could be.

Elders know something about not-knowing, about living with uncertainty. Their growing numbers, combined with a deeper awareness of the moment, provides the surest indication that evolution is happening in a timely way. Elders reveal that, despite hours dark with uncertainty, the human spirit can be aroused to live fully. This is a gift of the darkness — an uncertain, initiatory opportunity.

Something extraordinary happens in the final stage of life. All the ups and downs, the losses and gains, the times of unbridled confidence and uncertain vulnerability: all come together. The human form of Life can be actualized, becoming more fully what it means to be human. This is a strange, delightful, and ultimately mysterious occurrence. I like the term ripening because it is active. Ripening connotes an achievement — a state of being ripe — but goes on to imply a furthering of the process, moving towards seed making. Ripeness is a phase of being, a step along a larger more mysterious way, which somehow is never done.

All of the initiations, hardships, luck, intention and serendipity come down to a being like none other — one more totally human. This is an ordinary miracle. Life knows how to do it, and does it regularly, despite us. Ripening just goes on.

Eerie shadows can bring disillusionment, but this is the end of Life, as we know it — and the dawning of Life, on its own terms. Exerting a gravitational pull, unlike anything that comes earlier, this force, Life, this natural phenomenon, enters, bringing age marks, the wounds of loss, and the scars of hardship. These are honors, that temper and arouse character; greeted at first, as tragic indications that one is entering into decline. Whereas, on Life's terms — the first signs of elderhood are appearing.

The appearance of the third moon signals the most thorough and substantial change that Life has in store for the human organism. Ripe elders deliver a timely message to us all about the real complexity of being human. In this dark age, this is a bright possibility, one we can no longer afford to misinterpret, misunderstand, and ignore.

Life evolved us, for reasons we can only guess, and isn't finished using us, for its benefit. Our actualization serves Creation. The ultimate reason remains a mystery, but our very existence reveals that we are somehow a part of the whole. Our ripening is part of a larger ripening of Life. Life quests on, evolution proceeds, the Great Mystery unfolds and ripens us.

STAGES

As every flower fades and as all youth
Departs, so life at every stage,
So every virtue, so our grasp of truth,
Blooms in its day and may not last forever.
Since life may summon us at every age
Be ready, heart, for parting, new endeavor,
Be ready bravely and without remorse
To find new light that old ties cannot give.
In all beginnings dwells a magic force
For guarding us and helping us to live.

Serenely let us move to distant places
And let no sentiments of home detain us.
The Cosmic Spirit seeks not to restrain us
But lifts us stage by stage to wider spaces.
If we accept a home of our own making,
Familiar habit makes for indolence.
We must prepare for parting and leave-taking
Or else remain the slaves to permanence.

Even the hour of our death may send
Us speeding on to fresh and newer spaces,
And life may summon us to newer races.
So be it, heart: bid farewell without end.

—Herman Hesse

Section Two

2

. . .

THE TAO OF LATER LIFE

SEED

Some seed in me,
Some troublous birth, Like an awkward awakening, stirs into
life.

Terrible and instinctive It touches my guts.

I fear and resist it,
Crouch down on my norms, a man's Patent assurances.

I don't know its nature.
I have no term for it.
I cannot see its shape.

But, there, inscrutable,
Just underground,
Is the long-avoided latency.

Like the mushrooms in the oak wood,
Where the high-sloped mountain
Benches the sea,

When the faint rains of November
Damp down the duff,
Wakening their spores---

Like them,
Gross, thick and compelling,
What I fear and desire
Pokes up its head.

—*William Everson*

Introduction

Section 2 – The Tao of Later Life

I thought I was dying. I'd been living as a terminal patient for a long frustrating time (3 years) and expected to pass away at any moment. I'd started writing, in my one-handed way, using the keyboard as best I could, in a desperate attempt to avoid taking regret to my grave.

The writing brought me back to life. Literally and figuratively. Out of that desperate time came many things. I wrote that I would like to work with old people. My experience with stroke hardship, led to an innocent curiosity about aging. I had an idea that maybe the old, by virtue of their long lives, and the many hardships they experience— might arrive at the farthest reaches of human consciousness.

Years later, I helped found The Elder Salon, where I, and several dozen old folks, began a prolonged inquiry into the nature of getting old in America. Surprisingly, we discovered that we were not over the hill, as many people assumed, but more alive with growth and development than previously thought. We had inner lives.

I became fascinated, and began seeing that nature had created some people who kept on growing, and exceeded the normal cultural expectations for old people. Life seemed to follow patterns that impacted elder life. Something, very different than I had been led to believe, was happening.

The Tao of Later Life is a description of an alternative way of seeing later life, an attempt to give Life its due, by paying attention to what nature is doing, rather than going along with cultural assumptions. Life has cooked up an unexpected development that changes the way the latter phase of life is seen, and begs for attention.

Throughout this text the reader is going to be exposed to a confusing, but important distinction. Life, capitalized, stands for the evolutionary force. Whereas, life uncapitalized, stands for the personal years, which comprise the life cycle of any individual. One is of universal origin and ubiquitous, the other is shaped by the attitudes we embody.

The movement I witnessed had no explanation, appeared nowhere in the literature, and offered a very different picture of human existence. What I observed was deeply disturbing. The landscape I thought I knew became something else. Unintentionally, I was drafted by Life, to become a chronicler.

The thing that upended me the most, was the naturalness of what I observed. By that I mean that what happened was organic, arising unbidden, without anyone's intention. Life was propelling a shift — as profound and as natural as a pubescent human acquiring hair — marking the flowering of an inner life. A change takes place that is very different from the one that most of us had been led to expect. Nature is preparing a different outcome from the one that is socially assumed. Life places some kind of seed within. And this seed ripens into awareness.

Some old people carry a latency that alters them and adds fresh meaning to what it means to be human. I don't understand why, and can only speculate about some unknown process of natural selection. Nevertheless, it is quite remarkable to observe Life doing something unexpected. All of this action is happening within, just as externally it appears as if the body is breaking down.

I believe that without a name this important phase of human life would remain misunderstood, invisible and underappreciated. Grandolescence (see chapter 2 of Section 1—*The Evolving Elder*), is my way of describing signs of change in the older human organism. This phenomenon resembles closely enough the notion of spiritual growth to be conflated with it.

I don't claim to know what death is, nor do I have a notion of "afterlife," but what I have observed does suggest some kind of preparation. In the past I have seen this as an evolutionary process, the advent of a new kind of elder (see Section 1 — *The Evolving Elder* for more description). What I want to emphasize now, is the role of Nature—of Life itself—as being behind these changes.

Life naturally prompts the development of this internal being; through the difficulties and challenges usually associated with the later stages of life. Certain beings go through several differing phases during their life cycles. The mosquito, for instance, goes through three distinct phases: larval, pupal and adult. The first two stages take place in water, and the last in air. It could be that humans, in the bodies we know, represent only the early phases of development. There may be more to come. Such a complex organism might take multiple stages to grow.

Since the work of Jean Piaget in the 50's and 60's it has been widely held that children and young adults go through distinct stages of development. More recently, since the 1960's, developmental scientists have identified 8 to 10 (depending on the differing models) distinct stages of adult development. Cross-cultural studies have verified that human growth goes through a stage-progression, no matter the cultural context. There seems to be some biological component to this progression.

Although science recognizes the fact of human development, it has not as yet established a driving force. I believe it is Life's design that orchestrates the movements in later life. What I hope to reveal in these pages is that Life not only has designed human life to include unknown growth potential, but also provides naturally the prompts for it.

I have heard people talk about death as a kind of birth, when they (people) are thinking in spiritual terms, they view death as a move of the spirit from one life to another. I see a similar transition, but

I don't think of that shift as primarily spiritual. I tend to consider what's happening as a natural unfolding. Life is an incubator. It provides a holding environment, which both supports and stimulates growth.

Thinking of later life as *an evolutionary force* is an idea that has been heretofore overlooked. It is time to recognize the naturalness of this forward urge. That means thinking of the complexities, hardships, break-downs, and realizations that make up later life as tailored naturally. These difficulties draw out of us the sensitivities and awareness that prepare us for what inevitably follows.

Herein is a description of the events of later life—the circumstances that make that latter part of the human journey such a feared, misunderstood and incredible time. Essentially, old age isn't really old. It's a stage along the way, a sadly misunderstood phase of life. There are aspects of later life (i.e. old age) that transform consciousness, alter awareness and prepare us for an important transition. These elements of Life are not seen in the light I shine on them. *The Tao of Later Life* sparks another, better sensitized, look at what goes on in the later years.

Chapter 10
THE END OF THE STORY

S
ome say that death is the end of the story, but it may not be the end of the line. As our bodies run out of energy, break down, and end their service, something is happening, something that looks like what we have been led to expect, but which is quite different than what we anticipate. Nature, it turns out, has other plans for us.

What is presented herein is an alternative view of Life that alters perception and begins a new inquiry into an old phenomenon. The premises that follow are based upon careful observations of old age, the time leading up to the final scene. Until now, there has not been a sufficient attempt to look through the eyes of Nature. It turns out, that if one looks at old age, through eyes edified by Nature, a different perspective emerges. Life is up to something more than typically imagined.

I'm not exactly sure when the changes begin. Maybe, there is something always there. Inside. I have spent some time with friends exploring our first recollections of something strange going on within. For me, it took the form of dreams and strange synchronies, for others it was sensations, knowings, and guidance. In each case, something was palpable enough that it galvanized attention, and eventually led to a focus inward.

Late life is dominated by the growth and development of these internal sensations. Nature makes sure of it. Old people seem to be losing their faculties, becoming less and less functional, and while that is happening some are simultaneously being stimulated within, and becoming more attuned to a changing consciousness.

Interestingly enough, this phenomenon is not happening in defiance of aging—becoming more aware despite getting older—but becoming differently aware, *because* of getting older. Life is working them over. This falloff in capacity is an aspect of aging, widely perceived but less obvious, mainly because what's happening within is so remarkable: the old person is being altered. This change is so widely unexpected that it gets misunderstood and misinterpreted. Later Life alters consciousness.

In fact, losing and gaining is the pattern that Life uses. The loss is typically easier to perceive because it fits more into our cultural expectations, and generally happens externally. Much of the assumption of aging as decline is attributable to how readily perceived the loss aspect of older life is. Whereas the gain that always accompanies loss is not so easily perceived, because it is going on inside, where it is invisible.

This element of late life is easy to perceive—along with the challenges of a broken-down body — come new feelings and sensations. Feelings, such as increased awareness of how precious relationships are, a renewed appreciation of life, wonder, greater sensitivity, and a depth of awareness. Life breaks open some old people, and provides a different perspective.

Nature runs a paradoxical number on us human beings. Currently, the old are mainly feared, segregated, and avoided. Science dismisses them as over the hill, and religion too often treats them as children, who need to be helped to die. Something much more compelling and interesting is going on. Life, the biological underpinning of human existence, is preparing some of us humans for another form.

This assertion flies in the face of traditional assumptions. What I want to describe is so different from mainstream awareness, and so important, that it deserves to be expressed fully. Nature has designed something that defies our expectations, and takes us into realms of experience, that we are not prepared for. That is both the good and the bad news.

Life has devised, what looks like a way of aging us, while at the same time, putting us through a regimen of loss and gain that alters us. In an organic way, Life prepares us for death, and whatever is beyond it. This happens so naturally that we humans, with our deep antipathy towards death and old age, have failed to notice it.

The truth is that old age changes human consciousness more thoroughly than anything else. Hallucinogens pale beside the constant and totally idiosyncratic ministrations of the aging process. Aging breaks folks open by virtue of the many challenges it presents. Life penetrates the body, altering the mind, undermining the bulkhead of identity, and grooming us for what is to come.

Old age leaves one naked, helpless and uncertain. One gets to be around for the indignities. The chagrin one might feel about this inevitability is transformed by the realization that Life is priming one for a new form. Traditionally, this transition has been thought of as spiritual—but careful observation suggests it is metamorphosis, biologically going from one form to another.

The caterpillar melts down in the chrysalis in order for a butterfly to emerge. Just like it, a person breaks down through aging, and shifts to another, as yet unknown, form. What is most daunting is the fact that breaking down includes a loss of identity. One is no longer what one once was. This is one of the hallmarks of aging that has traditionally caused a lot of fear and apprehension, and interestingly enough, is considered an essential component of many spiritual traditions. The giving-up of identity is considered vital for the realization of a richer, wider, more sensitive and broad life. Life diminishes us, and thusly, grows us.

There are many occurrences of the death/rebirth cycle in a typical life. People go through a lot of rough spots, where their lives are radically changed by job loss, relocation, accident, illness, death of loved ones, or some other rite of passage. The kind of forced growth that Life generates is unwelcome, often seen as tragic, and is amazingly transformative.

As we are being reduced, we are being grown. Death and birth are oc-curring at the same time. The breakdown and the breakthrough are simultaneous. The overwhelming loss of functioning in one world frustrates in specific ways, producing a new, and different blossom-ing. This pattern, which has been observed everywhere in Life, is universal. It applies to us, sending our kind into the unknown. As we are dying, we are being re-made.

This makes the journey of life, a complex amalgam of adventures, which serve as transformative way-stations, temporary stops, that shape us, altering our nature, and increasing our viability. Life is a larger cycle, one that grows, ripens, and transforms us. Ageing inhib-its what used to serve, while developing what will now serve. The outmoded and antiquated, is built upon—the new emerges from the old.

From this perspective, it is pretty easy to see where the world's spir-itual traditions have originated. Each of them, in their own way, cap-tures something of the movements of Life. I'm not interested here in their relationships with power, ideology, culture and history. I just want to point out that Life's movement, a free, ubiquitously available, and always active source of transformation, is currently shaping our lives.

There is a new life that emerges as the old life passes away. It is not an "afterlife" per se, although it is partially composed of what came before; this is a new form of life. This emergence occurs as one is passing, not at the exact moment of death, but throughout the process of breaking down. Old age transforms, while Life cultivates, what it has placed within. Ripening occurs, bringing a passage into being, and catalyzing a transformation, that is to be looked forward to. This is ancient good news—though now it is complicated by mis-understanding, prejudice, and assumptions.

Old age may not, in fact, be old age. The body is breaking down. But we don't say the pupa is at the end of its life-cycle, we don't claim it is old, even though hatching out means leaving its bodily-form behind. A newer, more mature creature is emerging—even adopting a new media. Maturity may have to be redefined. This emergence is pre-planned by something beyond our assumptions, that has natural tendencies, something that we can observe, though we don't under-stand it yet.

Breaking down is no fun, no matter what. Breaking down with no idea of what is happening is downright frightening. So, there is a ten-dency to believe the old ideas that everything is over, that living is only a thing of the past. This is the end of the story, for us individuals, and for society itself. Perhaps there is an "afterlife." I won't know, for sure, until I get there. Life uses a pattern of loss and gain, death and birth, to regenerate itself. The old gives way to the new.

Old age is, for some, a time of being broken open. As people grow old enough, they outgrow, literally age past, ideas about who they are —they just know they are not what they used to be. For a time, they are story-less, they have gone beyond the old ideas, and often the fa-miliar limitations that once defined them. As a result of having gone past their own story, and being stripped of the old patent ways of knowing themselves, they come closer to their unknown true nature.

It is during this period of ambiguous identity that they are most sus-ceptible to experiencing the unknown and being re-shaped. Imagine, if you will, that this interlude is gravity-less, a time of radical un-boundedness, a time of incredible availability. It is a transition-al moment, full of unbelievable potential. This is when emergence occurs, when what is within is realized as most substantial. This is when a pattern that has slowly been cultivated by Life, goes on-line.

This story-less time has a lot of virtues. The narrative that one has lived by becomes more pliable, and its tendency to define one is greatly diminished. Imagine that people who have suffered limitations by virtue of where they were born, the parents they did or did not have, how much money their family had, class status, or the way they were treated, now have an increased opportunity to define themselves anew.

In a move that many people feel ambivalent about, Life has stripped them of their familiar identities, and replaced them with a more plastic, pliable opportunity to exist on different terms. Issues that once were the stuff of therapy, are suddenly resolved, or become irrelevant, by virtue of Life changing the nature of identity.

The power of story is widely acknowledged. The majority of us humans are so defined by it, that the focus upon the impact of story is essential. But less known, is the power of no story, or soft story. This power is mostly available to the minority that have been stripped of what they have known.

This story-soft experience, of disidentification with what was, where one has the opportunity to define oneself for oneself, loosens up identity and reduces external cultural conditioning, rendering one more available to what is stirring within. By itself, this identity-free zone provides transformative energy, moving one closer to a totally different, more organic experience of what is.

Emergence is a multi-stream blossoming, one that becomes increasingly more likely, as life-altering streams converge. Story malleability changes one's perceptions, alters experience, sensitizes awareness, and increases the likelihood of a larger being emerging. Emergence isn't subject to the laws, and efforts, of mankind. There is no formula, just a reliance on natural providence. Aging, considered widely to be the end of the story, opens up the door, breaks some open, and delivers the unbidden boon.

Chapter 11
KOAN-FU

———

Much of what I want people to notice is guarded by Nature. Life has devised a way to reveal what follows, primarily to those who have undergone some experiential preparation for this viewpoint. Like parenting, one cannot really get what it is like to have a child, until one has a child.

So, when I say that Nature protects this secret, I am referring to the process by which some things get only truly known through experience. Ideas may start out as brain-related activities, but some of them, like paradoxical awareness, go further. They are experiential. Knowledge of them only becomes more substantial and meaningful through direct experience.

Paradox is something that becomes most available internally, and in later life. Thus, it is hard to really know paradoxical awareness. Those without the benefit of the experience are going to have a different sense of the phenomena I am describing, based upon their particular life experience. Paradoxical awareness isn't universal, and it descends on people more frequently later in life, and thusly, seems to most like a plausible or implausible possibility, rather than a rarely occurring development that happens with some people.

Old age — and particularly the death transformation preparing part of old age — is largely invisible, and hard to take seriously, until old age arrives. Then, suddenly a bunch of changes begin occurring, most of them unanticipated, and some of them misunderstood. Life surges through us, in a way that looks different than it is. While it looks like old people are breaking down, some of them, are breaking open. Life is working a miracle it has worked many times before, but this time, it is hard to see. Life cloaks this transformation, and makes it most visible to those who have been prepared.

This is how that preparation takes place. Life asks everybody the same questions, but everybody doesn't answer in the same manner. From the myriads of ways human beings choose to live, some are selected for the particular challenge associated with paradoxical awareness. This is not a reward for good behavior, winning some kind of race, or possessing the right kind of merit, it is a seemingly random act of Nature that isn't really random. A kind of basic training is about to take place, and only Life knows what it is selecting for. Essentially, one gets drafted into a new more complex situation.

The miracle I refer to above, is a version of the same one that gave radiance to you in your mother's womb. All throughout life, there have been similar moments, that nudged all of us, onto the variety of paths that have defined our lives. Life has had its way with us, often without our notice, and despite our desperate assertions of will, control, and intention.

A select number of individuals, are drafted by Life, to be put through an initiatory experience, that changes their consciousness, into something that connects the opposites. These people don't volunteer — they seem to bumble naturally — into becoming aware in no way they intended to be. Paradoxical awareness seems to be Life's way of making its complexity simple. And, these few, are somehow chosen, to have that experience. A new encounter with wholeness follows.

One doesn't just acquire a new outlook. Instead, a bunch of new challenges, promote a deepening awareness, an unbidden sensitization, a disturbing view, a new perception of the relationship between things. The cumulative effect of all this stimulus, assails the mind, leading one into a newer place. An alien fogginess comes over the initiate, things aren't what they once were — and a fresh clarity starts emerging — the world starts looking, and operating, differently.

This change of awareness isn't something one seeks. The mind-altering elements of Life, gradually convert the mind. A pretty linear observance, gives way to more systemic perspective. Things that were once discrete, eventually, appear linked.

There is no easy way to characterize an age-related transformation of consciousness. Especially one that is unanticipated (thus seeming unlikely), and that does not take place in any kind of consistent manner. Paradoxical thinking, by virtue of its non-linear nature, arrives indirectly. Logical rationality suddenly finds itself befriended by relationships. Nothing stands alone —and the world has a new depth.

Perhaps the best way to imagine the change in awareness that slowly takes hold, and the gradual deepening of perception, and the changing view of the world, that occurs, is to think of a dojo — a place where a philosophy, and a new way of life, is being taught. The word dojo hails from Asian societies. A dojo is the place where martial artists are trained. Over time, practitioners evolve through a belt ranking system, that is based on tests of ability. These tests often involve combat with others. Eventually one achieves a black belt, which denotes skillfulness. Aging has no such explicit signs, but does test one, and provokes special developments.

People age accidentally into a phase of life that functions like a dojo. During that phase they are presented with a variety of experiences, that are tailored (meaning that they promote and aid in idiosyncratic ways) a gradual shift in awareness. Life, the Master of this dojo, trains its occupants without ever revealing to them, that they are being trained. Life, is altering people, without their knowledge or consent. Life, meaning some aspect of the biological forbear of all living things, instinctively re-shapes us, and renders us— through the particular training hardships it imposes — aware in a new way.

Old people wander in. Qualified by their rudimentary awareness that they know enough, to know, they really don't know much. Koans, and less formal forms of natural paradox, begin to appear. Tasks take on a more complex, multi-dimensional quality. These undertakings ask for a more nuanced treatment. In addition to logic, or intuition, these circumstances cultivate a more contradictory and enigmatic perspective.

At first paradox just becomes more evident. When it happened to me, I was amazed by my perceptions. It seemed to me, I was being taught (by no one in particular) a new language. Unbidden, there came into my awareness, a new simpler, yet more complex, way of describing the events around me. It was as if someone was whispering to me in a foreign language, that I began understanding. I gained a kind of elevated awareness. I began to notice the presence of contradictions, discrepancies, and strange relationships.

Later, I realized that paradox was catching my attention. With that realization came a kind of knowing, not exactly an intuition, more like an awareness that a puzzle was, with diligence, now solvable. I began to look at things, especially relationships, to see what they might divulge. Now, I think it is important to emphasize, I had no idea any of this was possible, or meaningful. It was like finding out that, with practice, I could hear whole discussions, where once I only perceived sounds.

Time passed, in my case it was at least seven years. I say at least seven, because I don't know if the training is over, I know that I contain a new unexpected awareness, which I rely on, but I have no sense that I can turn it off or on. I am not in control of this development. I stress again, that it came to me like body hair appeared when I was an adolescent. There was no volition involved.

I've come to realize how important this development is to well-being. Both/and awareness in addition to either/or thinking has allowed me to see deeper into Life, and lately, has enabled me to hold contradictory perceptions together.

That has unlocked dimensions of experience I could experience no other way. This has two practical applications. One, I am now capable of holding opposites together, and seeing how they are interrelated. For instance, I can see that light exists because darkness does, but now, I also grasp that darkness is another form of light.

This benefit enables a complex awareness. Some old people, because of this awareness, are able to be happy in the midst of global demise. They can perceive the everyday miraculousness of life, at the same time, and with the same vividness, as they experience the everyday horror of life. Side by side, there is a new perception of an on-going relationship, that broadens one's experience, and adds to the meaning of connection. Life is freshly enchanted.

This kind of interdependent awareness allows happiness to persevere in the face of significant difficulties. The growth of this kind of sensitivity, the freshly enchanting nature of things, may account, in part, for the overall happiness of older people. In any case, the advent of this kind of awareness draws the world together into important new patterns. New perceptions, and new awareness abound, changing the nature of life.

This same new complex awareness has a second significant benefit. By allowing a fresh look at how things are linked, it is possible to see (not literally, but figuratively) relationships that were once invisible. The relationships between loss and gain, grief and praise, death and life, become more perceptible — and then they totally alter awareness. This is of particular importance to how aging is perceived. There is a link between external, physical demise, and internal gain. The visibility, and viability, of this growth isn't available to the typical either/or awareness.

Either/or awareness is reductionistic, meaning it only perceives part of the larger picture, and by collapsing a relationship into something less than it is, renders invisible important features of the whole. Paradoxical awareness reveals more of any phenomenon, and makes important connections explicit. To perceive the actual benefits of older age a more paradoxical view is necessary.

The training Life provides can help reveal the normally hidden potentials of later life. This training isn't available to everyone, Nature seems to be up to something that cannot be predicted, or described very thoroughly. Elsewhere (in *The Evolving Elder*) I have described the ways we humans have for delaying, and even stopping, the growth of such awareness. But, here, I want to affirm that this form of growth in awareness is not subject to human intention. This kind of development occurs because Life stimulates it, not because we humans make it happen.

Thousands of acorns fall from a single oak tree, and only a few germinate. Millions of sperm cells desperately make the swim in the ovaries, but only one enters the Ovum. The way of later life appears to be no different, there is an unknown lottery process. For some reason, known only to Life at this point, this process of selection takes place, and it enhances the species range of awareness.

This is part of the unknown nature of later life. It follows a larger pattern that is only discernable through the pattern itself. Life seems to adhere to the practice of growth by reduction, the practice of making more with less. Reduction is another aspect of the paradoxical way of later life, another shift, that makes more explicit the Tao of later life.

If one were to imagine, that early more youthful human life took place in a tidal flow, that was directed outward, then one might grasp the shift that is taking place. Early on, everything seems to take place outside, in a flow beyond one's reference point. The normal flow is outward. This orientation defines early life, leading to an external focus, and the assumption that things like safety, evil, power and belonging are all externally related. They have to do with fitting into a preexistent order. Life seems to be about reading the environment around one, and shaping it, to make it more congenial.

There is a reversal that takes place for some people. Later in life, a minority of folks (about a third) discover that the tide shifts. They are empowered by a recognition that within them lies the flow that best allows them to express themselves. They become more internally directed. For them, the values they select and hold internally, define their experience of life. They live more from the inside out, and see things like safety, evil and power and belonging as internal factors that are subject to their own influence. For them, Life seems to depend more upon reading themselves, and shaping their own capabilities, to make their lives more congenial.

Later in life (that's what this book is about), an even smaller minority (about 3% of the whole) begin to have an experience that is highly disorienting at first, but later changes the way everything is perceived. They begin discovering that the tide actually goes both ways at once, and it always has. They begin to grasp this newfound sensitivity, and realize there is a relationship between the internal and the external. Slowly, they begin to explore how all things are interrelated. They experience life with a new depth. Safety, evil, power and belonging all depend upon their opposites; risk, good, weakness and isolation. In later life, Life carries a more inclusive, more paradoxical, perspective that reveals the natural ways Life makes existence more congenial to we humans.

This shifting pattern of awareness, holds another larger significance: everything about life comes into a new focus, with a simplified, and more complex clarity. Later life, which alters our physicality, and our identity, simultaneously, delivers us to a more complete picture of what living entails. Life and Death are as interrelated as everything else, they reveal a passageway, the in-between, that is, the joining of this stage of life with the next.

This kind of awareness appears in later life. Starting with the challenging awareness that one knows enough, to know how little one knows — a host of paradoxical realizations follow. Life trains us in this new awareness. It becomes full-time. Examples like; the fear of loss is soothed by loss, letting go of the old self, leads to possession of a new self; the place of one's limitations is the place of one's possibilities; and, one must die before one dies in order to live fully. This change of awareness is compelling, energy-giving, poignant, and enchanting.

Life turns into something quite magical. There is a sense that one has entered a world that is contiguous with the one has always lived in, but now is enchanted — full of delights, miracles, and the unexpected. Some greater mystery is unfolding and it is inclusive of everything. The world opens in ways that increase one's gratitude, belonging, and attention.

This change is just one stream of a greater change that happens in later life. How it happens is different in each life. There are many different streams, and they don't come on-line simultaneously. Each arrive in their own time, via different avenues of experience, but they all portend, and are part of, a larger emergence.

Chapter 12

A NEW CLARITY

W ithout some paradoxical awareness, it's hard to get the major benefits of aging. The weariness, and heartbreak of a diminished body, and the advent of death and hardship, makes old age look bad. Life definitely changes. Wrinkles set in, one gets gray, the body weakens, and social discrimination follows. Living isn't what it used to be. Life's change, isn't toward inevitable decline, for some, it is into a new stage of growth and development, a period of preparation for a new life.

People are susceptible to the consensual perspective on old age and death, thus there is a tendency to miss an opportunity that is folded into this stage of life. We are mesmerized culturally by the losses of old age, and consequently overlook the gains. Later life holds the most important aspects of living — but these gains accompany such a thorough period of loss — and they occur inside, where they are un-noticed.

The change that old age brings is so substantial, and physically challenging, that it really is a new phase of the human experience. A partial explanation for how its potential has been missed, has to do with how unexpected it is. Just as individuals are discovering— they are not what they used to be — so the human race is discovering, aging isn't always what it has been traditionally.

The change is so dramatic, and so big, that a difficult transition accompanies it. Going from adulthood, with all of its cultural identifications, into the elder phase, where all of the former ways of identifying oneself are lost — is the greatest and hardest transition that people face. And, until recently, it is one that has been unknown (see Grandolescence, Chapter 2 of *The Evolving Elder*). The potential of our species is squandered —when we incorrectly equate physical losses with demise — and misunderstand the scale of what is coming to pass.

The journey from lively participant in all the elements of a productive life, into becoming a dead weight, that impedes production, is not, to most, a desirable shift. Economic, and cultural production give way, to aging, and a more invisible, harder to measure, internal yield begins taking place. A massive shift of identity occurs — one that is so thorough, and so disturbing, that it throws most people into confusion and shame. This is a transition that our society doesn't prepare us for, doesn't value, and doesn't support.

It is like Mission Impossible. But not to Nature. Becoming old, and at the same time, full of potential, isn't even on our cultural radar. Instead it is totally organic shift, a movement made by Life, to forward something of our nature.

The radical transition from a cultural and economic being to one that is original, and oriented in a totally different way, is a challenging prospect experienced as an involuntary make over. Life drags some of us away from the life we've known — into another one, that operates in ways formerly considered improbable.

Each human endures the transition in his or her own way. There isn't a consistent pattern of changes, that makes it possible to predict what is going to happen next, and how things are going to progress.

The lack of a consistent pattern is one of the reasons this transition has been unrecognized so long. The extensiveness of this transition accounts for the prejudices, judgement, and invisibility, that many old people experience. The illusion of human disconnection from Nature, that prevails in our science-based times is great enough, that old age suffers, and we miss what it holds for us.

The natural unfolding of we humans, especially in the latter stages of life, is subject to the same kind of environmental dysfunction as that we have heaped on our earthly home. Natural evolution has been treated through our expectations — in this case, as demise. The opportunity that later life presents, is missed, because it doesn't look like what we are prepared to see.

Nature has its own plans, that are not subject to our presumed limitations. It puts everybody through a process of rigorous testing, that frustrates, confuses, and pares away our enormous hubris leaving a more humble, vulnerable, and teachable human being. Aging is full of unsavory losses, that make it seem like a curse —Nature's bad joke imposed upon us —when in fact, Life is pruning us in preparation for new kind of existence.

An opportunity is arising — everyone goes through a rigorous paring — to make transformation possible for a few. In earlier writing, I described it, as a "through the looking glass" change. One moves involuntarily from being externally oriented, to an internal orientation, and for a few, onto a more interrelated view. There is an equally frustrating shift from doing to being. Along with these massive changes in perspective comes a host of losses, body changes, and shifts in memory, values, and friends. All in all, there is a loss of general functioning and energy.

All of these changes stir up feelings. Life puts one in a new place, in a different body. And basically, you are left on your own to figure out what happened to you. This could happen almost overnight, or it could take a long time. Years can pass. People get old differently, each in their own way, but the inevitable comes to all of us, eventually. Aging is disruptive, it breaks people open, and a few find a new life.

The changes I described above are fairly typical — unfortunately so are the usual responses. Demise and diminishment have, by conventional standards, set in —there isn't much to look forward to.

The expectation of going downhill, leads to exactly that. Research shows that people who have a positive image of aging tend to live longer, healthier lives than those who don't. That is what makes recognizing such a major transition so important. The difficulties are easier to endure, when they are made more meaningful. Beyond this transition, a new set of experiences, meanings and possibilities await. Accessing the terrain beyond has consequences, especially for the happiness of individual old people, and also for the well-being of humanity.

Grandolescence becomes most tangible to people when they begin to feel the burn of losing. Loss might first appear in a variety of ways, but for the average aging person, it is usually personal and emotionally expensive. From the loss of a job, or the loss of social prestige, looks, health, loved ones, financial comfort, and other difficulties, one enters a world of greater vulnerability and less control.

There is an "about face" that happens as one ages. Things, people and places disappear. A life of acquisition becomes a time of loss, and letting go. Early on, there is a kind of shock, around the vulnerability of loss, then comes the realization that loss is going to be a constant companion in this new era of life. Letting go is always painful, sometimes debilitating, and totally essential. Life is loosening up the things that keep one bound — a very materialistic reliance —that assumes that well-being resides in externalities.

There is a kind of "shedding" that occurs in later life, that is important, and that the transition from acquiring to losing, brings into awareness. The losses of grandolescence at first feel tragic, as in early life, but soon become common-place and predictable (Everything that can be lost will be). Losing, and letting go, are features of latter life, that morph, as one begins developing a paradoxical outlook. What once was solely painful and tragic, become freeing and educative. The pain of loss is soon joined by the wonder of gain.

This is when it is possible to experience reduction. The idea behind reduction goes back to cooking. A good cook will immediately recognize that reduction is a technique used to enhance the savory nature of a sauce. Paradoxically, one gets smaller, while becoming more.

Without a more paradoxical awareness, it is easy to get caught in the tragedy of loss, and miss the opportunity and potential that is being released. Again, there are myriads of ways this can happen, but the upshot is that there is a clarification of being, a strengthening of intention. Aging looks quite different, it loses some of its 'demise' prejudices, when one begins to recognize that loss and gain are intimately interrelated.

The dramatic shift from identifying, and valuing oneself, by external standards, to finding the meaning of one's life "within" oneself, takes a while to unfold. The speed of this transition involves many factors, most of which are not in anyone's personal control. Things like; how much success one has had in adulthood, how much one already has an inner life, how comfortable one is without control, the amount of change one has already embraced, how much trust one has in themselves, and the ease with change that is imposed by Life. This amount of change may well take years — and some significant re-thinking. It isn't comfortable, effortless, and easy. Yet, losing is natural, and coming to each of us, as surely as the air we breathe.

The loss that usually triggers the recognition — that one is no longer, who one once was — leads to a relationship with loss that is pervasive, on-going, and definitive. Losing becomes an important, undesirable fact of life.

Growing into the benefits of aging, means being subject to changing, while facing the losses that naturally occur. It is a de-stabilizing period, that overturns what has been valuable about the past, while one is being introduced to a new landscape.

Reduction dominates this new landscape. This can be tragic, as it is to the majority of we humans, making aging look very undesirable, OR loss can be paired with gain. External loses, look ominous and feel debilitating, but can be highly sensitizing, leading to internal gains in awareness and capability. Who one is —is highly susceptible to the attitude one meets these experiences with.

Life's pairing of loss with gain is just one of the wondrous discoveries that comes along with the advent of a paradoxical perspective. In this case, reduction converts loss into something entirely different; a passport to a more functional inner life. Losing becomes an opportunity— the way Life grooms one — for what is to follow. Loss maintains its poignancy, it still hurts, but the hurt is transformed by the inexplicable recognition of gain. Life is up to something that transcends expectations. Losing leads somewhere, pain leads to an unexpected development.

Hurting, is not only a result of loss, but it is also birth-pain. Inner life is blossoming — complexifying emotions, perspective, and a new softer identity — while simultaneously — clarifying and making simpler; values, possessions, and relationships. A natural fluidity takes over — the integration of impermanence, and the relinquishment of control — follow. One, under the influence of reduction, begins to lean in, to become more amenable, to see the opportunity associated with difficulties, hardships, and unexpected events. A new sense of expectancy arises.

The few who survive — and learn to thrive, during the rigorous, yet enabling features of this time of decline/growth — are prepped for a more radical awakening. They are prone to experience a clearer recognition of Life, and of their relationship with it. The qualities of this element of aging enable greater fluidity. This fluidity, contributes momentum to greater awareness.

Aging, via these circumstances, creates another stream. That development doesn't guarantee an emergence, but increases its likelihood. Remember, what is described here is Nature's action, it is the result of forces intrinsic to the aging process —none of the potential unleashed by Her behavior is man-made. She is up to something, that we humans can only guess at, and would benefit from, if we could only learn to honor and cooperate with Her.

Later life offers a way to become more, a shift to a higher octave, an increase in what it means to be a human on this Earth. Growing is always an ambivalent process. It contains losses, gains, and new responsibilities. We humans tend to equivocate — as we are doing now — through our ageist notions, but Life wants to go on. Later life offers that chance. Instead of treating that as the end of the story, a tragedy that needs amending, we could be embracing Life's movement, we could discover there is something else happening.

Chapter 13
HONING A SNOWFLAKE

———

Life turns us all into artists. Without any effort on our parts. Something inside us stirs. When this biologically driven process begins to unfold, it is usually viewed as problematic, because it undermines the relationships that were once so fitting. Growing, being stirred by what is within, often means disruption of friendships and family. Happily, or perhaps not so happily, life helps by doing its job, growing an original seed inside, widening the gap between what is emerging and what is here. Basically, artistry, deciding how to respond to internal agitation, is a natural outcome of living.

Being buffeted around by the emerging self isn't easy, especially in a cultural world that insists upon growth milestones it can understand. Life has a way of thrusting each of us beyond ourselves, ignoring our comfort zones, feeding on itself, and fomenting a miracle of creativity. People become themselves. They add to the diversity of life and demonstrate the way Creation moves through us. We are all part of that big stream.

Being artistic means learning to work with the raw materials life provides. The essential experiences, and their integration into works of great accomplishment, take time. The soup gets better as it is cooked. Humans become more idiosyncratic, more uniquely themselves, as they go through the passageways of life. Each of us ends up creating a life that expresses who we are. We can't help ourselves; we are inadvertent and very proficient artists.

Humans, unlike other artists, don't have to go around looking for inspiration. The presence of Mystery, makes it clear, that Creation continues anyway, through us. This makes us automatically Creation's agent, an element in the Great Unfolding, a vulnerable artist working with the raw materials of Life. This isn't a voluntary activity; rather, it is one of those, a person can't help but participate in. Life drafts us. Life supplies us with the experiences, and we make ourselves original and unique.

We are carriers of a thread of creativity that is as old as our species We get to be artists, turning our lives into original forms, becoming the snowflakes that make Creation such a vital, diverse and miraculous thing. Free choice for us, means that we get to sculpt what we choose with what we are given.

In other words, the impulse to create is born in us. It stirs like some strange seed inside each of us, and then we are faced with creating a life that somehow gives expression to this wild, unruly, unknown impulse. We are living agents of Creation, and we are flesh and blood experiments.

Creation forces our hand, but in exchange, it has given us the adaptive ability to really create. The freedom to create, to live out an artistic vision, a vision of our own wholeness, is a great gift. It comes with great responsibility and potential. Both are burdens that can be carried happily or tragically. The quality of our lives is determined and made by us.

Making, for we humans, is a daily occurrence. Despite ourselves, and strangely because of ourselves, we make day-to-day choices, that result in the sculpting of a life, an expression of Life on the move. Without much thought, or self-consciousness, each of us, dealing with all manner of hardships and successes, is carving out a life. The process of living gives us the opportunity, through the ups and downs, to become ourselves. Life — no matter where we are, whatever our circumstances, rich or poor, sickly or healthy — provides us with the raw materials. What we do with them is up to us.

We are in a flow. Most of us don't know it, most of the time, but we keep at it. Life goes on. Sometimes it feels like we are swimming under our own power. Sometimes it is clear that we are being buffeted around, by unknown forces. We are threatened, and sometimes knocked off our original course. Whatever the case, we are involved in the process of shaping an idiosyncratic life, of making something of our being, of taking this experiment in Creation a little further.

There is this big operatic production going on behind our lives, and most of the time it isn't very apparent to us. As far as most of us are concerned, this is just a place where we are struggling to eat, to have a steady roof over our heads, and to share with another what living brings. The flow of Creation is mundane and real. Each little act contributes to a broader pattern, a rivulet of Life, that ends up in a greater sea.

Sometimes the import of the moment, the circumstance that calls for self-definition (sculpting), are as clear and palpable as the rain; and sometimes, the moment when one's life changes, is as ephemeral as the moisture in the air. Just as water continues to flow through its cycle, Life continues to take shape, not only as an expression of our choices, but as a carrier of the experiences that help us form our choices.

We are Life's life. It creates us at the same moment we are living it out, giving it a particular shape. All of this flowing towards us goes on day and night, and whether we forget it, or never believe in it, it happens anyway. What we do with it is our artistry. Our particular lives are shaped, as existence teases out of us our unique response.

The flow of life experiences is our amniotic fluid. Within it we are created, and miraculously, we get to shape ourselves. The Universe, because it wants as much diversity as it wants unity, has invented some kind of paradoxical wizardry that enables humankind to be unique and part of the whole.

There is no escaping this flow. Each of us is composed of relationships, is involved in relationships, and is impacted by relationships. The tides generated by the gravitational pull of all things, buffet us around. As we go, we age and become ourselves, as we determine and meet the obstacles along our course, we create out of an endless sea of possibilities a unique response. Life has its way with us. We end up facing the unexpected. In the meantime, it is *the response* we generate which shapes us.

What we meet and what meets us interact. Out of this interaction, and most particularly out of our response, comes something that is uniquely an expression of ourselves. We are in this moment deciding how we want to respond. Sometimes the onslaught of challenging conditions seems like too much. Being in over our heads is a sure sign of being human, of existing, of the struggle of living. The painful, uncertain times rouse our creativity. The expansion of the Universe comes through us. How we respond is our business. Our lives are our own, but a larger being also has a stake. We choose the how, but we don't choose the what. Life thrives on us, and we thrive, when we live and shape ourselves accordingly.

The connected life holds a particular challenge that is especially relevant to the art of becoming true. By virtue of always being in the gravitational pull of relationship, it is hard to maintain a consistent shape. All of this relationship affects one. The degree to which relating affects and distorts one, bending one into a new shape, or reinforcing the inner resilience of one (staying true), depends upon maturity.

True expression, and the artistry it generates, benefits by relationship pressures. These pressures help define the self, and teach one how to maintain shape. The wants and needs of others can be overwhelming. Eventually these relationship forces necessitate a kind of growth. In order to not be run by the desire to please everyone, by taking their preferred shape, there comes a need to decide, to hold to a particular shape (to become one's self), to become someone instead of a shape shifter.

Early in life, this is a real character-building hardship. Always, throughout life, one is confronted by choice. Becoming oneself is a process of facing greater and greater pressures. Diamonds are made by being subjected to extreme geological pressures. The jewel that is each of us, also takes shape and becomes more solid under similar interpersonal pressures.

Life helps. It serves up the salient, just-right, relationship dilemmas. We are each blessed (sometimes it feels like a curse) by some kind of strangely unerring navigational system. We find our way, with Life's help, into and out of the relationships we need, to become more fully ourselves. This is a strangely elegant inelegant process. Sometimes it seems that despite ourselves we become ourselves. Life puts us right into the situations that require us to make choices that shape who we are.

Life never gives up on us. We are always being asked something. True creative expression is an ongoing thing, like a conversation, a kind of call and response. Maturity doesn't mean arriving at some final state of completeness. That isn't how Life works. True artistic expression is a process of becoming more and more true to the uniqueness emerging within.

There is a story going around, a popular but infuriating tale. The moral of this story is that one creates one's own reality. This is a compelling message, for two reasons, because it seems empowering, and because it contains some truth. The half-truth of this message implies that the Universe cooperates with all intentions all the time. Not so. manifesting is a collaborative process. The Universe has its own stakes.

The art of sculpting a self is one filled with intention, intention that navigates through the intentions of others. The art comes from being influenced by these diverse sources, while steering toward an intended outcome. The trick here, is not to arrive where one intended, unchanged by the process. The art is to go upon a creative journey where the end product is surprising — better because of the influence of others.

The help received along the way isn't always welcome. The Universe has an interest, it meddles, seeking its own agenda. Sometimes experiments have to fail. Obstacles appear. Hardships temper the process. Manifesting reaches a dead-end. Artists are thrown back upon themselves. These are the moments of doubt, that seem to authenticate the creative process. They are openings for inspiration, which always seems to come from some other source.

Manifesting is a non-linear kind of phenomenon. What manifests is often quite different from what is intended. This variation, this straying from the original vision, is a hallmark of creativity. The art of becoming, is some unpredictable combination of the intended with the unintended. The artistry comes naturally, through just trying to persist during the onslaught of raw materials (the flow) coming one's way. The art form of human life is some combination of our intentions with Life's intentions.

The Mystery that emerges from within, and becomes oneself, is really a residual component of The Big Bang. Out of nowhere came the Universe. Out of that same place comes the self. What we get to play with, what we get to be creative around, what we tend to call our own, isn't really ours. That which we call ourselves belongs to something we don't really understand or know. We are Life living its way into the Universe. It is very likely that we are extensions of the Universe. Manifesting a self is the Life's way of becoming more, expanding, playing out a drama that includes us. We ride the currents of that dramatic expansion, becoming ourselves, as our way of furthering it.

This fountain of creativity is one of the attributes of the Universe's ceaseless energy. This ongoing energy event, the Big Bang (still under scientific contention) is the greatest energy event, and the most creative occurrence ever known. The artistry of our lives is part of the continuum of Creation. This makes us offspring of something so big, powerful, and generative that there is lots of room for us to be innovative, to create our lives in totally unique ways. Being true to ourselves is being true to the Universe.

These lives are not just our own, we may do with them what we please, and whatever we do will serve Creation, but we further Creation best by paying attention to what we sculpt. We are creations of Life, and we serve the ongoing thrust of Creation. Our fate is tied to the whole. That is a kind of appropriate and just destiny. All we have to do is figure out how to live it out. We are given the raw materials, and we make of them what we can. Creation feeds on our artistry, the uniqueness that is each of our lives. Creation relies on us to extend its reach, to give it perspective and originality. The unique quality of each of our lives depends upon living up to the way the whole depends upon each of us.

Chapter 14
UNKNOWING

———

Like it or not, life has set things up so there are always more possibilities than any of us can imagine. We are adorned with more unknowing than we can easily handle. This is one of the existential facts of life, that is extremely elusive. The impact of it (unknowing) is unpredictable. It is a wild card in the deck. It makes the game, which can go any direction, a game of chance. Our lives revolve around not-knowing, around being at the mercy of mysterious conditions, that provide unpredictable surprises. Life, as one famous artist said, is what happens to us, when we are making other plans. Not-knowing shapes us in ways we cannot predict, but must respond to.

Some say, "Life is unfair." It is true, there is this seemingly random thing, something that is throwing a major monkey wrench into all of our ideas about how life should go. This is one of the most predictable aspects of the unpredictability of our lives. There is so much we don't know. Unknowing reigns — from the time and means of our death, to the chances of making it from here to there — we don't know. It is all a crapshoot, and we have to make a life without knowing what each moment may bring.

Humans are vulnerable to the unknown, to what seems to be random, to ambiguous forces beyond us. This is a fact of our existence. Uncertainty is inconvenient, messing with all our plans, and liberating us from our ruts. Unknowing, like it or not, plays a major role in our lives, shaping us in unpredictable ways and forming who we are.

Serendipity is always at play. This fact, that we really don't know what is going to unfold, is both a gift and a curse. The element of uncertainty plays a role in our development, and gives us the ability to respond creatively. Time unfolds us, that is true, but not-knowing challenges us to hold onto ourselves through the storms of good and bad luck. The pattern of who we are, that which distinguishes us, undergoes a lot of unforeseen changes, that knock us into and out of shape, and can serve to help us realize what endures, what is true about us. Uncertainty leads us to be more certain.

How can one build castles of any sort in the surf of constant change? Well, the answer that seems to be the preferred response is try to pretend that uncertainty doesn't exist, that the quicksand isn't really a feature of this life. The surf, after all, only comes occasionally. Everyone is subject to not-knowing, but early on, most people try to pretend it only happens to others.

It is easy to see why. Uncertainty is overwhelming. Why start any endeavor if it is likely to veer off in some other direction? It is better, and seems more possible, if one just ignores the likelihood that change, the unpredictable-ness of life is going to intervene. Blind faith is not the same as audacity. But early on, pretending that life will cooperate has an appeal. And that appeal is primarily an illusion of control.

The sense of being in some kind of control is far more reassuring, even though that sense is inaccurate. We really don't get to know how things are going to turn out, or even by what process stuff is going to happen. Notice how unappealing that idea is. Human life, my life, must be on some kind of stable footing! I rely on so many things; my partner, job, home, location, family and friends. Who am I, if all of that, or any of it, changes? Really grasping how little I really know creates in me a terrible feeling of vulnerability.

For that reason, I like science, technology and games. They appeal to my desire for order, for something I can predict, for something I can rely on. The particularities of my desire to have something to rely on, my desire for the illusion of control, are not important to this essay. What is important is that you recognize the bulwarks you have put in place to protect you from your own vulnerability before uncertainty.

My choices — science, technology and games — reflect my attempts to escape what I don't know. Science, with its restricted factors, control groups, and reliable, repeatable outcomes, calms me down. I've learned to see scientific results as interesting, but not as accurate. Technology gives me the illusion of control. I rely upon mechanisms to give me a sense of the predictable, even though I complain about the arbitrariness with which they seem to work. I like games too. Rules circumscribe game reality and give me a momentary feeling of things adding up. I like to win. For a while I get to have a sense that I am really competent.

Then reality returns. Typically, when it does, the door of consciousness is kept closed. The fact of not-knowing, of being at the mercy of the unknown, is so undermining that most of us don't let that awareness in. Why should we? Isn't it better to find some way of operating that can be relied upon? In the early stages of life, unknowing is seen more as a debilitation, something to be overcome. This is an indication of how much pressure there is to conform, to find a way to fit in, to create a life that works, literally as well as figuratively.

Giving in to unknowing, refusing to proceed into the unknown, these are choices that are just not acceptable early on. Pretending that we do know, and can know; that is more acceptable. Reality is what we pretend it is, isn't it? We don't get to know. That isn't in the plans. But, there it is; uncertainty, never-the-less. There is so much emphasis placed upon not being stopped by uncertainty, that people are oblivious to what uncertainty introduces into our lives.

Unknowing is sort of like the monster in the closet. It doesn't really exist, except it does. As we age and get more experienced, uncertainty grows. This is usually an unwelcome development. The monster of unknowing comes out of the closet, and the horrible realization that we live at the mercy of something else comes with it. As much as we scramble to put our heads back under the covers, it is difficult to shake the recognition that life isn't what we thought (pretended) it was. The monster demands recognition.

When enough of our plans go awry, and we stop blaming ourselves, or others, then we begin to notice that life seems to work differently than we had been led to believe. This is a painfully horrible, and ultimately liberating realization. Uncertainty, like it, or not, has a place at the table. Coming to terms with what you cannot understand or even anticipate, is part of life.

There are many strange discoveries that accompany a life. Amongst the strangest, and oddly most surprising, is the discovery that not-knowing is a friend. How can this be? So many years have been spent warding off this encroaching realization. Even so, getting the full impact of not-knowing isn't assured. Experiences stack up, the predictable life falls down, and some people recognize that they have to surrender to the fact that they are not in control. Aging, because it brings more experience, convinces us. The old saying that "the only constant is change," is true.

The truth is that unknowing doesn't grow; we do. There is no more unlikelihood now then there was then. What there is, is more appreciation for how changeable, how unpredictable, how unknown everything important is. Life, by throwing us screwball after screwball, has softened us up. The experience of being off balance — and knowing one is off balance — becomes too overwhelming to ignore. Balance becomes a much sought after capacity; and as it does, the unknown becomes a more real experience. In fact, one begins to realize that balance seems to hinge on the soft, ever-changing nature of what is not known.

As the awareness of the depth of unknowing dawns, so does the capacity to begin accepting and coming to terms with it. The presence of uncertainty, unknowingness, grows us. There is a change that takes place as one begins to see the pattern of not knowing that underlies human life. This change occurs as the self ripens.

There is a paradox that lives at the heart of unknowing. The more you live, the more you become aware of how little you know. Unknowing is like the monster come out of the closet — now it seems to be everywhere, and it is changing life. The changes themselves are more uncertain.

There is this strange feeling of being made more solid by what you don't know, and more permeable, at the same time. Balance no longer seems to be a steady thing; it is more like a constantly moving, fluid kind of thing. What you don't know may not kill you, but it is likely to alter your trajectory. The dynamics of the moment are no longer straightforward. Life, it seems, now has a life of its own. The unknown creeps in, and creates a whole different kind of human being; uncertainty has this strange ability to generate a sensitivity to the moment.

This is the beginning of a new relationship with being. This new beginning takes you down the rabbit hole. It introduces you to a world that is fluid, changing, and where things are not just what they seem. This "through the looking glass" reality is closer to home. Proportion shifts. The world is full of strange new possibilities, and you must make use of some of them if you are going to be real.

Uncertainty turns us around. It introduces us first to probability, then to not knowing, and the deeper vulnerability that, like death, means that things can change in an instant, and that nothing about life is predictable. This softens us up, and prepares us for living more deliberately. When everything can go or change instantly, one becomes prepared to be creative. Unknowing turns us all, like it or not, into artists. We create lives that are subject to the moment.

Long ago (in the 18ᵗʰ century) a French mathematician created a model that captures the paradox that lies at the heart unknowing. He pointed out that if all knowledge formed a sphere, then when knowledge grew, so grew the surface area of the sphere. What this meant, was that as the sphere of knowledge grew, its surface came into greater contact with the unknown.

As we grow, as we know and experience more, we come into contact with more of the unknown, and it seems that we know even less. The unknown hasn't increased, but our contact with it has. The world we live in is more alive with uncertainty because we have grown, and now we have a greater chance to become beings that are familiar with the unknown. This changes everything. When Mystery dawns; the world comes alive in a new way. When we no longer know, we become more available to learn.

There is an ancient assumption that old people are privy to wisdom. There are two forms of wisdom; the known and the unknown. The older one is, the greater the likelihood, that one has gone through the kind of experiences, that imparts wisdom. Known wisdom is based on experience, is rooted in the past, and is predictable. Unknown wisdom is new, rooted in the present and future, and unpredictable.

Unknown wisdom, if you will, is 'wiser wisdom' derived from the unknown, and only available to those who are comfortable with not-knowing. Old folks give access to both, but only those who have been stripped of their certainty, humbled by the recognition that they have no way of knowing, and have grown familiar with the underlying uncertainty that attends Life, have access to this rarer, harder to achieve, and less known, form of wisdom.

There is a poignancy to not-knowing that characterizes the elder experience. Humility rides shotgun with uncertainty. There is no such thing as expertise, no identity that comes with not knowing, just a reverent openness. Openness is essential, enabling Mystery to have an impact, life to be what it is, instead of somebody's hope.

There is a stream of awareness that emanates from unknowing. It is a kind of innocence that is unlike the innocence of childhood. Instead of ignorance, the unknowing described here, is a deliberate awareness, a kind of surrender, a reverence for a larger un-comprehended reality. Humbleness and openness characterize this stream of awareness. They deepen over time, and contribute to a greater awakening.

Unknowingness is characteristic of late life development. Not-knowing is the way many old people are. They aren't demented, and aren't suffering from some other form of addled thinking, instead they have a handle on the true nature of reality. Life is festooned with uncertainty. The Mystery that haunts and defines the moment is always disguised. Life has seen to it, and some old people have become in tune with it.

Out of unknowing, out of an appropriately blind engagement, comes the kind of openness from which some new possibility is born. Something unknown, unseen, unexpected, gloriously unusual emerges. The future rests on the new and unique. Emergence makes the implicit explicit, it takes humanity into realms humans have not knowingly occupied previously.

Chapter 15
EMANCIPATED INNOCENCE

There is a wide-open state of mind that is incredibly compelling, practically mesmerizing, and at the same time, gullible, naïve and excruciatingly available. This is a highly prized capacity— that can easily be viewed as a tragic vulnerability. It comes later in life, and can be preyed upon by the unscrupulous, or be the source for a very rare form of wisdom. It is a state of mind that is totally guileless. It is admired, feared, and accompanies some in later life.

Innocence involves a guilelessness, that characterizes early life, and disappears throughout adult life, until it is restored by an amazing act of shedding, pulled off unwittingly. Life restores innocence by administering a coup de grace — that is so profound and complete — that it takes away all bearings. We call it death. But it is not the final exit — just an advanced portion of dying.

Innocence in late life — unlike in the life of a child — is a by-product of loss. It is being thrust beyond the gravitational pull of all that is known, and all that has called one. It is a state of existential nakedness. Weightless and naked, beyond all artifice, there is a portion of human life that is seminal. It isn't new, though it has never existed before. In childhood, it came around expressed as magical fascination. But in elderhood, to a minority of folks, innocence comes around again, as a bout of fascination that has been freed from all outside influence. From it, creation ensues.

Like all rawness, there are efforts to cover it up, to protect it from abuse, or less innocent use — this rawness exists — because Nature has deemed it important. Innocence has a place in Life that is essential. It isn't just childish folly, or an old person's silliness — it is the way life introduces novelty.

That's why people get hypnotized when there is a baby present. Something magical can happen — and it's all natural. Life is encountering the way things are. And as we all know; things aren't always what we think they are. Innocence provides a fresh take on reality. It is the way we humans experience what is — naturally— without the intercession of others.

Innocence is more than 'not knowing,' or experiencing something for the first time. There is a willingness to engage. This willingness to join, goes far beyond the fear of the unknown, which is learned. Life embraces Life. Naturally, innocence entails a rare greeting, that informs, integrates, and absorbs. Mystery is treated as a friend.

It is hard for the culturally-influenced mind to even imagine a state like innocence. For good reason. Innocence is not man made. It occurs only when Nature has introduced pure mind to what is. Usually this happens twice in human life; through infant naivete, and elder emancipation. Each represents a kind of purity; the guilelessness of a child, and the freedom from influence won by the liberated elder. There are important similarities, and important distinctions. The emergence that innocence enables hinges upon those differences.

Childhood innocence distinguishes early life. It demarcates the onset of awareness in a wonderful way. The encounter with reality is utterly fresh. There is no mitigating force, no intermediary, at the beginning. Everything has a kind of glowing neutrality, a magnetism all its own, an attraction that is untainted and genuinely vivid. Mothers know that this curious engagement can be dangerous, so they are always close-by. To the infant, all is wonder. It is this attitude, practically a total demeanor of wonder, which makes infants so beguiling, and their first time encounters so interesting.

Right away, both consciously and unconsciously, the people environment, especially the parents, start transmitting attitudes, beliefs, and prejudices.

Innocence goes on, well into early childhood, but cultural reality soon eliminates it. Innocence gives way to a particular knowing, that others transmit to help make one safe, secure, and part of what's going on — for belonging's sake. As a child develops and becomes an adult, innocence gives way to this knowing. The child takes his or her place in the reality of family, community, and culture.

The openness of childhood wonder is so amazing to see. It brings with it a mix of feelings, from awe to envy, but usually some form of nostalgia for the loss of the unmitigated experience of the world. The usual assumption, is that natural marveling is past, never to return. Adulthood is not as free, experimental, creative, and unbounded. It is as if one puts on a garment that grows rigid over time. One can easily get trapped, becoming predictable, less vital, and boring.

Happily, for many old people innocence returns. The rigid garment of old assumptions and expectations passes. A new sense of wonder comes on, in an unexpected way, and is frequently misperceived. So, the benefits are often missed. Old folks are privy to a wonder of Nature, that is unknown to most younger people.

Younger people are so entrenched — in their adherence to social norms — that they are unable to entertain the idea that something new and different could be occurring. Early on, the freshly old, tend to maintain the blind ideas that run in the conventional mind. Resisting, and categorizing ageing, they do not see the possibilities inherent in this stage of life. Elder innocence initially lies under a blanket of assumptions, that obscure it, and tend to pathologize its signs — as cognitive impairment, dementia, feeble-mindedness, or anything else — besides what it is.

Elder innocence is something else, something so adaptive and powerful it offers a transformative possibility. By virtue of the process of loss, the old person is shorn of all their reference points, all the reliable ways they have known themselves, and reality. They evolve into an experience, whereby, they are not at all what they used to be. A natural pruning happens.

Along with the onset, or exacerbation, of ailments, a natural period of reduction occurs, where Nature takes away all of the elements that once so reliably defined them. Slowly, often quite painfully, they lose not only functioning, but friends, family, capabilities, mobility, and sociability. They are reduced. They are stripped of memory and acuteness, but they retain the capacity to experience things again, for another first time.

Trimmed of the non-essential — which once seemed so essential — some of the old become available to Life in a way they only knew in childhood. Without the old familiar reference points, they are free to have totally idiosyncratic responses to what they meet. The moment becomes electric with possibility. Each encounter is new, unfabricated, pristine, and rawly charged with the unknown. This is an elderhood that is rare, pregnant with possibility, and totally a product of Nature.

It is also an opening, a rarefied aperture, a gateway of sorts. Each of the streams of loss provide the altering power that shifts everything. Innocence peels away the superficial and gives access to the depths of Mystery. This is the ground from which the essentially new emerges.

Now, it is possible to grasp what is so liberating and important about elder innocence. It portends an unknown future. There is, inherent in it, a knowing embrace of the unknown. The openness that characterizes this element of life, pretty much guarantees an encounter with what is. Reality becomes real like it almost never is. Suddenly, the range of the human organism is extended.

This is one of the essential ingredients of evolution. There is no guarantee that a greater emergence is going to come through this organic expectancy, but there is an increased likelihood. The potency of first contact permeates each moment, bringing with it a vibrancy that enlivens and enthralls. Innocence like this is a lightning rod, it draws energy from the environment.

A growing prospect of greater emergence is potentiated, but just as Ben Franklin sent the kite into the air, he still had to wait for lightening to strike to discover electricity — human beings must wait for Nature to strike. Innocence optimizes the conditions, but emergence happens when it will. Change is always happening, in big and little forms, the trick is to recognize that which changes everything. Elder innocence empowers little changes, and welcomes bigger changes, when they appear.

Innocence alone can bring about a fabulous new level of awareness. When this unknowing combines with the other streams then a river of possibility is unleashed. Then emergence of the new is made much more likely, then a torrent of change promises to sweep us into the future, then the next stage is much more likely to become palpable.

Chapter 17
OPENNESS/EMERGENCE

———

L ife has conspired with Mystery to create some kind of weird turnaround. While physical wilting is setting in, something new is stirring inside. I've never been as alive as I am right now. Youth isn't wasted on the young, unless, aging is wasted on the old. Life seems to ignore that waste, in favor of a crop of those living anew with uncertainty.

We have forgotten what we once knew. Life doesn't begin, or end, with us. Some strange aliveness, a few would call it 'a second childhood,' a new life, is besetting some old folks, and changing the meaning of being fully human. As our bodies head toward becoming inert, some seed in us, is nearing lift-off.

It may be strange to think that there is a potency, a kind of latent life-force, that resides in, and is only perceptible, in a place, that has been considered the end of life. It may seem contrary to everything one has been taught about life, but it's happening anyway. Life is more than we humans have thought it was. Humanity has failed to look past its assumptions, and see a bigger, more accurate picture.

One of the values of getting older is the capacity to perceive life again, to gain new perspective, to see patterns one could not see at earlier stages of life. There are traits that come on, that are embellished by, the radical losses that accompany later life. Without experiential knowledge of loss and gain, it is too easy to overlook the formation of something, that remains, when it seems that all is lost. Paradoxically, our greatest loss is that we don't perceive our greatest gain.

Meanwhile, Life keeps churning. The tides set-off by the life-force keep fomenting change, altering the path, adding new dilemmas and opportunities, growing us, sometimes overwhelming us, all without our knowledge (and consent). Life moves us toward some mysterious occurrence, that we fail to acknowledge. Getting old, entering latter life, is when Life comes rushing into awareness, just as the truly old rushes out. Losing creates space.

There is something about the losses, the emptying out, the slow diminishment of energy, that enables mystery to take place. This is an organic part of being human. Our animal nature has us participating in the dance of birth and death, creation and destruction, renewal and expiration, departure and arrival — that is the way of Life. Later life makes this reality more explicit. The way (the Tao) of later life, is acceptance of the dance — and of one's place within it.

Humans have intuited the Tao for a long time. Throughout the ages, wherever culture evolved, and became stable enough, practices and perspectives appeared, that tried to capture the mysteries of existence. A careful reading of human history reveals an on-going inquiry into the Cosmos— internal and external. This inquiry is taking another turn, it is going beyond where it has gone before, it is manifesting in a new energy released by Nature. Human life expectancy has grown — and now — for some, that means experiencing Life as never before.

The primary assertion of this text is that in the later years of human life a change takes place, that is widely unanticipated, misperceived, and is fundamentally benign. As death approaches, for some people, the way it approaches, sets off a cascade of losses, that paradoxically prepare one for the emergence of a new life form.

This is not, per se, a spiritual journey, set off by some kind of deity, life of intention, or appropriate practice, rather, this is the work of Life. It happens no matter what. What is amazing, and I hope evident throughout this treatise, is that Nature has created naturally a process of moving from external orientation toward an inward one — that is fed, and nurtured by — the stripping of all the physical and psychological components of one's former life. In the later years, what becomes apparent, is that throughout life, a living force, a natural phenomenon, has been steering, interfering, and aiding the emergence and ripening of fresh possibility.

The world's spiritual traditions have had a great civilizing effect upon our long slog toward greater awareness. They cannot be honored enough. Now, however, it is possible to see how much they have relied on a kind of bio-mimicry, to further their work — they have designed theology, and practices, that were closely aligned with the actions of Life. They have recognized from their perspective, what is now evident from a more modern perspective. Life takes away the unnecessary.

Part of the difficulty often expressed by the ageing person, especially in those years between adulthood and elderhood (the grandolescent time) is the sense that identity is shifting. Many people express it as, "I'm not who I used to be." This feeling grows more and more vivid as one ages. Later life contains a radical shift. Everything by which one has identified themselves, starts to disappear. Live long enough (which is happening now), and everything melts away.

The being that is left has been stripped of all the trappings of identity. They are devoid of the earmarks that convey a place in society — they are bereft of the fundamental things that make them an identifiable being. A baby's lack of identity, is comparable to the loss of identity, that takes place in later life. A baby comes in a pretty blank being, an older person near their end, is someone who has been stripped of the non-essential. Each moves forward; one naively dispossessed, gaining weight, and the other unburdened, and gaining lightness.

If one considers the typical trajectory of the old, it becomes fairly obvious that they are gradually stripped of the ways they have been somebody. If they live long enough, Life removes the chaff and leaves an essential kernel. This is a time in life when the story is less definitive and compelling. Not-knowing grows. And innocence and paradox enchant the world. Any of the streams of change that are natural in late life, hold the potential to break one open. Being shorn of a life-story is a hugely enabling loss. When openness comes into the foreground, then emergence grows much more likely.

Much of the stripping that takes place near the end of life isn't all that personal —some of it is social. Life tends to take some people beyond the gravitational pull of mass mind. All the referent points— cultural, political, status, privilege, and attachments — vanish before the existential cleaner. Loss is an equal opportunity happening. It doesn't recognize cultural boundaries. Everyone, eventually experiences their lives avalanching into oblivion.

When falling takes place, there isn't anything to hold onto. If one didn't know it before, then one learns, that impermanence is a promise Life keeps with ruthless impeccability. The habitual has no immunity. A lifelong pattern of assumption passes too. Innocence is all that survives. Emptying out, one passes into clarity, no longer blinded by what used to be.

The necessity of escaping from the conditioning of a life lived in a certain way, often at the behest of the past, is clearly an important pre-condition for experiencing something new. The masters have known this for a long time. Even before there was any idea of being available to the new, Life was practiced at getting rid of, or using in new ways, what no longer served. Emergence comes when the way is clear. Soft story, unknowing, and innocence clear the way — they don't make it happen — but they do increase the chances.

Not-knowing is a threshold to vastness. Added to that, is the paradox of later life; what is, is best discovered through what is not. Letting go, the pervasive surrendering that comes with aging, empties one out, allowing a space where Mystery can thrive. Absence, the loss of what was, opens up the opportunity for the new. Engaging the unknown, is in late life, something one does unbidden, without a choice, surrendering is just the way things go. Openness is just what's left when everything else goes.

This is not a quality of intention. Stripping takes place, and is so precise and exact, because Nature takes away all that one identifies with, not to be mean, but to prepare one for baptism into a new reality. It is said that Nature abhors a vacuum, but more true, is that Nature creates a vacuum, so it can be filled anew. Openness sucks, drawing in, what resides in the unknown.

It seems like at the center of human existence, like at the center of the galaxy, there sometimes resides a profound emptiness. Like a black hole, exerting a huge gravitational pull, the core of our being seems to focus inward towards a great absence. Absence prepares the way, gobbling all light, all knowing, and all hope. Only the new and unknown survives. What remains, or is truly original, can only become palpable when all else is removed.

Openness is a precursor that enables discovery, but precedes it with a natural aching for fullness. The loss of one aspect of life prepares the way for another. That is why openness is so extolled by spiritual teachers, who often are great observers of Life.

There is a line in a poem by William Everson that goes like this, "There is nothing so humbling as acceptance." When one is floored by the magnitude of awe, that is generated by the ache of emptiness, the potency of what's missing, the force of absence is strong, it can humiliate and humble.

There are larger powers that buffet, shape, and define us. Not just for our sake. This becomes more obvious to some in later life. When Life reveals a larger reality, a purpose beyond our pedestrian assumptions, a greater being, then a re-adjustment begins to take place. Perspective sets in. When acceptance overtakes one, humility follows.

Humility reflects a recognition of context. It is a fluid virtue. Required for learning, humility is the best attitude for meeting the unknown. It is an allowing, assenting, recognizing, bowing force. Humility is compliant with what is. It gives admittance to the unknown. Humility has long been valued as perhaps the truest sign of realization. It is an attitude that dawns when the shades are pulled.

All the stripping, forgetting, and loss, that comes with later life has a paradoxical effect. It prepares one for a brand-new encounter with Life. There is much more of a sense of being embedded within a larger entity. Paradoxical awareness enchants, and gathers reality into a larger, more energetic and vital world. Unknowing allows it to be something unknown and surprising. Life becomes a miracle that cannot be foreseen, but is enjoyed.

Just as unknowing sets in, and becomes stronger, an experience of familiarity grows. One is known, while growing more unknowing. This is a realm that doesn't adhere to the usual laws of science. Interdependence, connection, mutuality, relationship and belonging are the usual traits of this way of being. Later life takes on potential that is only found in the rarest accounts of hermits, monks, and exotic philosophers like Lao-tzu. This state of vibrant potential, defined by what is not there as much as by what is — is a product of Nature that helps direct us towards metamorphosis.

The basic theme of this treatise is that later life contains the essential ingredients that prepare we humans for the next stage in our growth. The experiences of later life, are often regarded as painful and debilitating, because they tend to strip away all of the accoutrements of a former life. What is mainly unknown and unrecognized, is that a new being cleansed of the nonessential, now moves into the light. This one is lighter, more conscious, and flexible in new and creative ways. What seemed like an ending has morphed into another beginning.

No one can say what form this new beginning takes. Metamorphosis at this level is typically unexpected. It is reasonable to expect uniqueness, but no one can predict the nature of the unknown Mystery that is unfolding. Emergence follows no pattern, adheres to no hope, cannot be expected, yet happens anyway, according to some drum beat of its own. Life goes on, using death, or what looks and feels like the end, to propagate new life. The end is the beginning. Newness comes through oldness.

Loss begets gain, just as compost renders the soil fertile. The radical remake that occurs as ageing breaks down the body, enabling a whole new being to emerge, not as a baby, but as a maturing, and better adapted organism. Death contains seeds. Life thrives, through what passes. Impermanence is a gift, that allows Creation to proceed. The losses of later life, are the raw materials, the enabling precursors, the amniotic fluid, that contains and energizes what is to come.

Life is essentially mysterious. It came out of the processes of the Universe. Science cannot really account for the metamorphosis that took place long ago: when the non-organic became organic, and life began. It is part of our species unknowing. We would like to pretend that we understand: scientific theories help perpetuate the illusion that we do, or can know eventually. But, the truth is that Mystery runs beyond our beliefs. Life is so much bigger than our assumptions.

I'm put in mind of an experience I recently learned about. A friend reported on watching his infant grandson learning how to operate his body. The child was reaching out for an object that had caught his attention. My friend observed how this small being organized himself in an effort to touch, and eventually grip, the desired object. Reaching was full of trial and error. It took time, and a major commitment of energy.

Repeated failure led the little being to discover how to coordinate and operate parts of his body. Through the whole process, it was fascination and desire that powered his changing capabilities. Life endowed this little uncoordinated mass with the desire that organized his efforts and eventually allowed him to achieve his goal. As my friend observed, "Life actualized itself."

Without any self-conscious effort, Life is carrying us into the unknown. We are reaching, or more appropriately one might say, Life is reaching, using what remains of us, to fulfill its desire. It is taking away what now is superfluous, preparing us for the next round of creative adventure. The preparation hurts, it involves loss, and less obvious gain, and finally the stopping of one form of life. This is how Creation proceeds. It reaches for a new form. Humans get to be made over. It is a poignant, beautiful dance, full of pathos, miracles and ultimately unknowing. Life goes on, the dance carries it forward, as paradoxically, Life carries the dance forward. Reaching, reaching, reaching....

Annotated Bibliography
(compiled by David "Lucky" Goff, 9/21)

* twelve recommended readings

1 — aging
2 — activism
3 — death
4 — spirituality
5 — evolution

What Are Old People For?, Dr. William Thomas, VanderWyk & Burnham, 2004
An excellent book for its time, it describes some of the benefits of aging, to old people and society alike. This is a good read for those who have an interest in promoting the needs of old people. Unfortunately, this book leaves out any description of the fears and rigors associated with the transition from adulthood to elderhood. It also fails to make an adequate distinction between the merely old and elders.

Second Wind: Navigating The Passage To A Slower, Deeper, And More Connected Life, Dr. William Thomas, Simon & Shuster, 2014
Here the author takes a sociological slant upon elder development and ageism, recounting some of the historical divisions that make-up American society. This is a thought-provoking approach. The book urges us to slow down, and take the ending of adulthood seriously. This is useful, but really misses the humanness (the existential aspects) of aging.

*1 —Life Gets Better: The Unexpected Pleasures of Getting Old, Wendy Lustbader, Tarcher Penguin, 2011
She is a geriatric social worker who beautifully portrays the value of older life, telling very real and poignant stories. She has a great capacity to portray the difficulty and beauty of senior life. But, she leaves out

any developmental perspective, and any general description of that age cohort. She does, however, demonstrate how the elder perspective could be useful to younger people.

*1, 3 —The December Project, Davidson & Schachter, HarperCollins, 2014
This is a report of the thoughts and actions of one of the most controversial and thought-provoking elder of our time, Rabbi Zalman Schacter-Shalomi This book suffers from an exclusive focus upon him, and poorly describes the rigors and advantages of elder life. It is nevertheless thought-provoking and an educative read, especially for those touched by his courageous efforts to keep growth and development on the map for old people.

*4 —From Age-ing to Sage-ing: A Profound New Vision For Growing Older, Rabbi Zalman Schachter-Shalomi, Warner Books, 1995
This book provides an important description of the spiritual and psychological benefits of aging. A forerunner in the field, that has served many people interested in having a rewarding and growthful late life. This book offers little recognition of the difficulty of transition from adulthood. Nor, does it offer any evolutionary perspective on aging now. It is, however, the prime read for those who want to contribute in later life.

The Age of Actualization, Goff & Hart, self-published, (available thru Amazon) 2014
This book is extremely useful in validating elder development, and in growing a sense of connection amongst elders. The book is focused primarily on the creation of elder community, but it does a really good job of portraying the positive benefits of getting older. The authors have experience with elder community and demonstrate why it is important to elder development. They also offer a bunch of vignettes to help people start an elder's community.

Growing Older, David "Lucky" Goff, self-published, 2015
This book reveals a more positive attitude about aging, and therein provides a valuable service. It is well-written, and brings home the

actual experience one has as they get older. It focuses most on the surprises that accompany aging, describing the attributes of the second half of life. He does not, in this work, discuss the opportunities associated with aging sufficiently.

*5 —The Evolving Elder: Applying What Really Matters to Life, David "Lucky" Goff, Ph.D., Eldership Academy Press, 2017
The author is an evolutionist, who sees the longevity revolution combining with an extraordinary ageing demographic, as Nature's response to the human adventure. This book contextualizes age-related developments, as part of an evolutionary thrust. It is beautifully written, and contains the author's initiation by hardships of Life.

*1,4 —The Second Half of Life: Opening The Eight Gates Of Wisdom, Angeles Arrien, Sounds True, 2005
This is a beautiful work, which is designed to promote important thinking about the developmental issues associated with a good life. It is a very stimulating work, which is good for use in a group. The book is laid out in such a way that it promotes introspection and sharing. It fails to describe societal benefits of aging, and totally leaves out the rigors of the transition to elderhood in our culture.

*1,2 —The Making Of An Elder Culture: Reflections On The Future Of America's Most Audacious Generation, Theodore Roszak, New Society Publishers, 2009
This is the seminal work on the topic of the coming of age of the baby boomers. It is a more demanding read, but it offers a very valuable perspective. While the book has much to recommend it, it is too speculative, political and suffers from an early elder's activist orientation.

* 1. —In The Ever After, Allan B. Chinen, Chiron Books, 1989
The only book thus far published that takes a cross-cultural look at the phenomenon of aging. It is poignant and an entertaining read. The stories are rich with particularly elder dilemmas and developments. The book offers a rich perspective with many metaphors that provide insight into elder dilemmas. Unfortunately, this book suffers from an exclusively psycho-spiritual perspective, which includes some very technical language.

1 —60 On Up: The Truth About Aging In America, Lillian B. Rubin, Beacon Press, 2007
This book is one of the most accessible books on aging, is topically written, and totally misses the big picture of development. The book is very accessible and well written. It makes clear that aging isn't what it used to be. It is one of the only books that takes on elder relationships as a discrete phenomenon. There is unfortunately no attempt to offer a view of aging as an evolutionary phenomenon.

1, 5 —The Creative Age: Awakening Human Potential In The Second Half of Life, Gene D. Cohen M.D., Ph.D., Avon Books, 2000
An exploration of the nexus between ageing and creativity. This book gives ageing a good name. It looks at the ageing's creative potential, and encourages self-expression, growth and relationship. The book is relentlessly positive, favoring creativity, but overlooking the many challenges that older people face. There is no other book that shines a constant light upon the creative attributes of a lifetime of experience and awareness.

*1, 5 —The Mature Mind: The Positive Power Of The Aging Brain, Gene Cohen, M.D., Ph.D., Basic Books, 2005
This is a major contribution to the field that focuses primarily on brain science. His work was the first that contained references to developments in brain research that showed the older brain in a good light. He is very positive about elder development. The book suffers, in my opinion, by providing little insight into the societal and personal benefits of the elder life stage.

*4 —The Gift Of Years: Growing Older Gracefully, Joan Chitchester, Bluebridge Publishers, 2008
A beautiful book that reveals one woman's reflection upon the benefits of aging. This is a beautifully reflective work. It highlights a positive attitude and demonstrates the sense of enchantment that is possible in later life. This wonderful perspective provides no societal insight, which can contribute to the aging process being something that can serve in a larger way.

The Art Of Aging: A Doctor's Prescription For Well-Being, Sherwin B. Nuland, Random House, 2007
A very apt and able description of the physical changes that accompany aging. A good read. It is encouraging, but fails to adequately address meaning, on the personal and societal level. Nor, does it attempt to address the evolutionary implications of this phenomenon.

1,5 —Gerotranscendence: A Developmental Theory Of Positive Aging, Lars Tornstam, Springer Publishing Company, 2005
This book is an important, even breakthrough, study of elder awareness. Read it if you really want to grasp something of the potential of elder consciousness. While the author provides valuable evidence of the potentials associated with aging, this work suffers in obscurity, and is written in the technical language of an academic sociologist, whose second language is English.

*3,4 —Still Here: Embracing Ageing, Changing and Dying, Ram Dass, Ph.D., Springhill Publishing, 2001
This is a book about the spiritual implications of aging. He is a disabled author who has been the light of his generation. He grasps something about the spiritual nature of later life. This book is inspiring, but it suffers from focusing exclusively upon the travails of its author, and does not really look at aging generally. Still, it is highly provocative.

*1 —Travels With Epicurus: A Journey To A Greek Island In Search Of A Fulfilled Life, Daniel Klein, Penguin Books, 2014
This is a delightful book, full of philosophical reflections on ageing, fulfillment, and the daunting task, that most older people face, that is, creating a philosophy to live later life by. Daniel writes in a very accessible manner, and emphasizes throughout this work, the great power of pleasure, literally of making the best of life. The emphasis on friendship, community, and conversation is refreshing.

*1, 3,5 —Paradoxes of Our Final Years, Elizabeth Bugenthal, Ph.D., Elders Academy Press, 2008
A beautifully written appreciation of later life, especially the change of consciousness that comes then. She captures the way wholeness grows

more evident with the onset of a more paradoxical form of awareness, and how Life becomes more poignant and miraculous as community with others grows. Her surprise and pleasure about what old age offers is our surprise and delight.

Naked At Our Age: Talking Outloud About Senior Sex, Joan Price, Seal Press, 2011
A book about the sexual nature of some senior relationships. This is a taboo topic that is handled lightly. Intimacy may be the most important thing to old people but that doesn't mean heat and desire have to be abandoned. This book is as hot as we are. This book speaks especially well, about women's sexuality, without demeaning men.

Triumphs of Experience: The Men of The Harvard Grant Story, George E. Vaillant, Ph.D., Harvard University Press, 2012
Faithfully following a group of male Harvard graduates throughout their lifespan, this longitudinal study reveals how much age can impact identity, self-worth, values and relationship. The sample is all male, white and privileged, but has the benefit of showing that ageing is an equal opportunity occurrence.

The Blue Zones: 9 Lessons For Living Longer, Dan Buettner, National Geographic Society, 2008
Through a great deal of cross-cultural research, the author is able to identify the essential components of a long, happy and healthy life. What makes this work stand-out is that the author places as much value on social connection as diet. It is good to know that centenarians are the fastest growing part of the age demographic, and there are places in the world, where local culture, enables elders to thrive and contribute. There is much we can learn from them.

*1, 2 —Happiness Is A Choice You Make: Lessons From A Year Among, The Oldest Old, John Leland, Sarah Crichton Books, 2018
He is a journalist for the New York Times. He takes the reader along as he discovers, through the lives of 6 old people, that happiness is not dependent upon material well-being, but the spirit and wisdom of age.

This is an inspiring book, that lets these elders speak for themselves. He writes well; the book is surprising, informing and inspiring.

*1, —The Measure Of My Days; One Woman's Vivid, Enduring Celebration Of Life, Florida Scott-Maxwell, Penguin Books, 1968
One of very few such books written by someone in their 80's. She has many interesting things to say about ageing. One of the most interesting facets of what she has to say is not what she says, but how she says it. She is an early example of the way consciousness changes with age. She exhibits a more paradoxical take on later life. It is important to note that she had already exceeded the life-expectancy of her time. That makes her insights remarkable. A short, very readable book.

Fruitful Aging: Finding The Gold In The Golden Years, Tom Pinkson, Ph.D.,self
-published, 2012
This is a wondrous book, containing a lot of indigenous wisdom. Tom is a healer, trained by the Huichol, and applying that kind of sensitivity to the growth and honoring of elders in Marin County. The idea, and practice, of Recognition Rituals is startling, an initiation of responsibility for greying individual and community alike.

Contemplative Aging: A Way Of Being In Later Life, Edmund Sherman, Gordian Knots, 2010
An early pioneer who recognized that late in life there is a move inward towards the powerful pull of an inner life. In addition to exploring the action-less side of life, his book is full of encouragement for practices that make this side of life more palpable. This is a relatively easy read for such a challenging, and ultimately rewarding topic.

4 —Spirituality and Aging, Robert C. Atchley, Ph.D., Johns Hopkins University Press, 2010
A timely book for those interested in the spiritual repercussions of living. He provides an extensive perspective on a very sensitive topic area. He writes about what spiritual experience are, to spiritual elderhood, and on into the sociological implications of a spiritual life. His work covers issues like death, grief, spiritual resilience and joy.

*1,3,5 —Sky Above Clouds: Finding Our Way Through Creativity, Aging, and Illness, Wendy L. Miller and Gene D. Cohen, Oxford University Press, 2016
Sky Above Clouds tells the inside story of how attitude, community, creativity, and love shape a life, with or without health, even to our dying. Cohen and Miller draw deeply on their own lessons learned as they struggle through aging, illness, and loss within their own family and eventually Cohen›s own untimely death. What happens when the expert on aging begins to age? And what happens when the therapist who helps others cope with illness and loss is forced to confront her own responses to these experiences? The result is a richly informative and emotional journey of growth.

*1,2 —This Chair Rocks: A Manifesto Against Agism, Ashton Applewhite, Celeton Books, 2019
Her disbelief and anger are infectious, especially if one begins to take in the amount of carnage this prejudice causes. She faces it head on, and even finds it within herself. She asks important questions, and offers important history and insights. This is a landmark book that makes visible a form of bigotry that has been socially acceptable, until she shines a light on it.

Centenarians: The Bonus Years, Lynn Peters Adler, J.D., Health Press, 1995

Celebrate 100: Centenarian Secret to Success in Business, Steve Franklin PhD. And Lynn Peters Adler, J.D., Wiley, 2011

The Book of Elders; The Life Stories & Wisdom of Great American Indians, as told to Sandy Johnson & Photographed by Dan Budnik, HarperCollins, 1994

Acknowledgements

How does one acknowledge Mystery?

I was born a normal human child, unaware that I was also being cared for by an invisible force. Then, this unknown force set me on a course that led to this writing. I didn't know I was headed this way. I don't think my life is predetermined, but it surely is influenced, in no way I can imagine. From the sublimely small details, to the agonizing choices a life is composed of, I was steered without any awareness, to a maddening desire to try and give voice to Life's role in our lives. All that truly qualifies me for providing these ideas, is the twisted trail that led me here. So, I'm inclined to acknowledge the unknown, and how it creeps into everything unnoticed. Considering the contents of this missive, I am just glad, that who knows what, blows this way.

There were people who helped too. From the grandfather describing the miraculous movements of his grandbaby, to the life coach who gave up on me, and said, "Write if you must." I was as assisted by doubters, people who couldn't see what I did, as much, as by those who encouraged me. What came through me here is everyone's, or no one's. It was written by me, but the contents aren't mine. Mainly, those who helped were the ones who loved me enough to care for me while I wandered in writing delirium.

The relative coherence of what appears in this writing owes itself to the integrity of what is coming through. I guess one has to be as isolated and disabled as I am, to have the time to experience the amazement of existence's secret. Now, it's a secret that is out, and depends upon other acts of Life to come to be known. A few of my most ardent friends read the text an offered editing suggestions. Although I will not mention their names, I feel how much I appreciate and honor their efforts. Mystery knows more about how this tract came to pass, and who to credit, than I do. And Mystery will more aptly acknowledge them than I will.

About the Author

David "Lucky" Goff, Ph.D., M.F.T., served as adjunct faculty at the Institute of Transpersonal Psychology (Sofia University), where he employed large group processes to promote community and personal development. David also assists organizations, including therapeutic and spiritual communities, in their quests to create and sustain genuine community. His research into the "psychological sense of community" is the first to examine and describe the conditions that facilitate collective consciousness.

In 2003 David had a brain aneurism. As a result of his stroke, and the onset of a rare brain syndrome, he nearly died and ended up permanently disabled. This experience had a transformational effect on David, which made him "Lucky," and cued him into how radically connected all things are. This broader awareness now informs his approach toward what it means to be human.

He maintains a psychotherapy practice specializing in psycho-spiritual development. He also writes extensively about a psychology of interdependence (see *Embracing Life: Toward A Psychology Of Interdependence*), learning community, elders and the conditions that lead to a social and ecological experience of connection. He can be reached at dg1140@sonic.net.